Steen Kølvraa

The Syndrome of D-Glyceric Acidemia with Hyperglycinemia

AARHUS UNIVERSITY PRESS

AARHUS UNIVERSITY PRESS
Aarhus University
DK-8000 Aarhus C, Denmark

Denne afhandling er i forbindelse med nedenstående tidligere publicerede afhandlinger af det lægevidenskabelige fakultet ved Aarhus Universitet antaget til offentligt at forsvares for den medicinske doktorgrad.

Aarhus Universitet, den 1 marts 1988.
Gorm Danscher
Dekan

The present review is based on the following publications:

1. S. Kølvraa, K. Rasmussen and N.J. Brandt: D-glyceric acidemia. Biochemical studies in a new syndrome. Pediatr. Res. *11*, 825, 1976.

2. S. Kølvraa: Inhibition of the glycine cleavage system by branched chain amino acid metabolites. Pediatr. Res. *13*, 889, 1979.

3. S. Kølvraa, N.J. Brandt and E. Christensen: Non-ketotic hyperglycinemia. Clinical, biochemical and therapeutic aspects. Acta Pediatr. Scand. *68*, 629, 1979.

4. S. Kølvraa, E. Christensen and N.J. Brandt: Studies of the glycine metabolism in a patient with D-glyceric acidemia and hyperglycinemia. Pediatr. Res. *14*, 1029, 1980.

5. S. Kølvraa, N. Gregersen and N.J. Brandt: Excretion of short-chain N-acylglycines in the urine of a patient with D-glyceric acidemia. Clin. Chim. Acta *106*, 215, 1980.

6. P.B. Mortensen, S. Kølvraa and E. Christensen. Inhibition of the glycine cleavage system, hyperglycinemia and hyperglycinuria caused by valproic acid. Epilepsia *21*, 563, 1980.

7. S. Kølvraa, F. Rosleff and N.J. Brandt: Normal glycine transport in cultured diploid fibroblasts from hyperglycinemic subjects. J. of Inherited Metabolic Disease, *6*, 82, 1983.

8. S. Kølvraa, N. Gregersen and E. Christensen: *In vivo* studies on the metabolic derangement in a patient with D-glyceric acidemia and hyperglycinemia. J. of Inherited Metabolic Disorders, *7*, 49, 1984.

9. N. Gregersen, S. Kølvraa, P.B. Mortensen: Acyl-CoA:glycine N-acyltransferase: *In vitro* studies on the glycine conjugation of straight- and branched-chained acyl-CoA-esters in human liver. Biochem. Med. and Metab. Biol. *35*, 210, 1986.

10. S. Kølvraa and N. Gregersen: Acyl-CoA: glycine N-acyltransferase: *In vitro* studies on the glycine conjugation of straight- and branched-chained acyl-CoA-esters in rat liver. Biochem. Med. and Metab. Biol. *36*, 98, 1986.

PREFACE

This review has been based on studies carried out over the periode 1974-1986 during appointments at the University Department of Clinical Chemistry, Aarhus Kommunehospital, Department of Pediatrics, University of Copenhagen, Rigshospitalet and Institute for Human Genetics, University of Aarhus.

A number of people have been helpful in the various stages of the projec I would like to express my gratitude to the following (in alphabetic order): Niels Jacob Brandt, Ernst Christensen, Bent Friis-Hansen, Niels Gregersen, Ida Grøn, Hanne Jacobsen, Rud. Keiding, Christian Knudsen, Inga Knudsen, Per B. Mortensen, Mette Houman Møller, Karsten Rasmussen, Flemming Rosleff, Sonja Rou, Dan Matthiasen and Vibeke Winter.

Financial support has during the years been granted by The Danish Medical Council and The University of Aarhus.

CONTENTS

II

1. INTRODUCTION

The application of sophisticated chromatographic and mass spectrometric techniques in the clinical laboratories has led to the discovery of numerous inherited metabolic diseases during the last decades. In most of these disorders the clinical symptomes are not specific. They are diagnosed by an extensive metabolite screening of the body fluids followed by a definite proof of the defect at the enzyme level.

In 1976, a seven-day old boy with severe hypotonia was refered for metabolic screening (Brandt et al., 1976; Kølvraa et al., 1976). Surprisingly, the results of the initial metabolic investigations suggested that this boy suffered from two different inborn errors of metabolism (i.e.o.m.). Firstly, the boy was found to have an excessive accumulation of glycine in all body fluids, most pronounced in the cerebrospinal fluid. This picture is typical of the syndrome nonketotic hyperglycinemia, which is a well known i.e.o.m. presenting with hypotonia in the neonatal period (Von Wendt, 1980). Secondly, the patient excreted substantial amounts of D-glyceric acid. This compound had not previously been found in elevated amounts in patients with nonketotic hyperglycinemia. It has however been found accumulated in two patients with neurological symptoms similar to our patient, but without hyperglycinemia (Grandgeorge, 1979; Duran et al., 1988), as well as in a patient with chronic acidosis, also without hyperglycinemia (Wadman et al., 1976).

From these data it is tempting to surmise, that the boy simultaneously suffered from two different i.e.o.m., namely "nonketotic hyperglycinemia" and "D-glyceric acidemia with cerebral dysfunction". However, certain amounts of caution over such a conclusion would be appropriate for the following reasons. Firstly, the probability of a boy having two rare i.e.o.m. at the same time is extremely unlikely. Furthermore, hyperglycinemia has previously been found associated with organic acid excretion, in connection with the accumulation of organic acids derived from the metabolism of branched-chain amino acids (Nyhan et al., 1972). This hyperglycinemia, which was previously called "ketotic hyperglycinemia", is now considered to be of secondary nature, and not due to an inborn defect in the metabolism of glycine. The possibility that the boy suffered from one single i.e.o.m. and that the other accumulation was a secondary phenomenon could therefore not be totally disregarded. However, with the existing knowledge about the metabolism of glycine and D-glyceric acid, it was not possible to formulate a single hypothesis that could explain both accumulations.

A number of tracer studies were therefore performed in order to elucidate whether a common defect lay behind both accumulations. At the same time each of the accumulations was investigated separately and the findings compared with what was known for syndromes with the same pattern of excretion. Tracer studies did not support a quantitative interrelationship between glycine and D-glyceric acid. From metabolic investigations it was concluded that the patient's glycine metabolism was identical to that found in the syndrome nonketotic hyperglycinemia (Kølvraa et al., 1979). Investigations on the etiology of the patient's D-glyceric acid accumulation were less conclusive, but suggested that the patient had a defect associated with fructose degradation. This finding shows the patient to differ at least from the most well-documented case of D-glyceric acidemia (Wadman et al. 1976).

The first set of data obtained thus seemed to indicate the existence of two different enzyme deficiencies with consequent accumulations in the same patient. Further investigations included a number of experiments aimed at finding a possible connection between the two enzyme dysfunctions. These investigations included in vivo studies on the patient, in vitro studies on cellular material from the patient and finally, model experiments on animal tissue.

The aim of the present review is to present the results achieved from our investigations of the patient with combined D-glyceric acidemia and nonketotic hyperglycinemia.

Firstly, the normal metabolism of D-glyceric acid is described - and against this background the existing cases of D-glyceric aciduria are discussed.

Next, the normal metabolism of glycine is considered, followed by a discussion of the various diseases associated with glycine accumulations in amounts comparable to those found in our patient.

The patient with hyper-D-glyceric acidemia and hyperglycinemia is then presented in detail. The data that elucidate the genesis of each of the accumulations and the data aimed at illuminating a possible connection between these accumulations are presented.

Finally, the review contains a number of considerations on whether the patient had a currently unknown i.e.o.m. causing both accumulations or had two different i.e.o.m. at the same time.

2. THE GLYCERIC ACIDEMIAS

2.1 THE NORMAL METABOLISM OF D-GLYCERIC ACID

Most studies on the metabolism of D-glyceric acid have been performed on liver tissue, and it has been shown that this compound participates in a number of reactions (Fig. 1). It is thus a component of the so-called non-phosphorylated pathway between serine and the glycolytic pathway at the level of 2-phosphoglycerate. In addition D-glycerate is a metabolite in the degradation of fructose.

2.1.1   The position of D-glyceric acid in the serine-glucose pathway

Serine is connected with the glycolytic pathway via two pathways: 1. the phosphorylated pathway connecting 3-phosphoglycerate with serine, via 3-phosphohydroxypyruvate and 3-phosphoserine (Pathway I) and 2. the nonphosphorylated pathway connecting 2-phosphoglycerate with serine, via D-glycerate and hydroxypyruvate (Pathway II) (Cheung *et al.*, 1969; Walsh and Sallach 1966). A number of researchers have investigated the relationship between these two parallel pathways. It has been shown in rats, that serine pyruvate aminotransferase (Rowsell *et al.*, 1969) and D-glycerate kinase (Kitagawa *et al.*, 1979) are induced by glyconeogenetic stimuli, and that D-glycerate dehydrogenase is feedback-inhibited by glycolytic intermediates (Kitagawa *et al.*, 1975 A). A gluconeogenetic role of pathway II is further supported by investigations on the pre- and postnatal development of the enzymes involved. In rats, it has been shown that both serine pyruvate aminotransferase and D-glycerate dehydrogenase are strongly induced at the time of birth. Maximum activities of these enzymes occur in the suckling period when gluconeogenesis from serine has been shown to be very high (Snell, 1980). Pathway II however seems more complicated. Studies on the intracellular localisation of the enzymes involved have shown that serine pyruvate aminotransferase is located almost exclusively intramitochondrially, while D-glycerate dehydrogenase is preferentially cytoplasmatic. Further, about 75% of the D-glycerate kinase is found within mitochondria and 25% in the cytosol (Kitagawa and Sugimoto, 1979). Finally, the glycolytic degradation is located in the cytosol. These observations seem to indicate an interrelationship between mitochondria and cytosol in the glyconeogenesis from serine. This interrelationship seems to involve mitochondrial transport of hydroxypyruvate, D-glycerate and 2-phosphoglycerate. However, nothing is known about the transport systems involved.

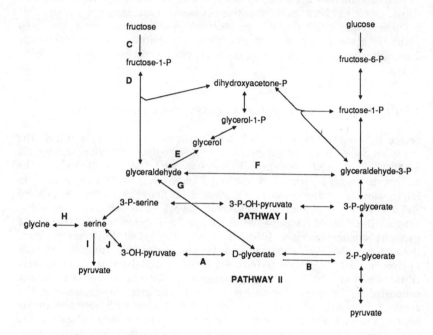

Fig. 1.   The normal metabolism of fructose and D-glyceric acid in liver
             tissue. A: D-glycerate dehydrogenase; B: D-glycerate kinase (very
             low in human liver); C: ketohexokinase; D: aldolase; E: alcohol
             dehydrogenase; F: triokinase; G: aldehyde dehydrogenase; H:
             serine hydroxymethyl transferase; I: serine hydratase; J: serine
             pyruvate aminotransferase.

The enzymes in pathway I react in an opposite manner to the enzymes in pathway II when given glyconeogenetic stimuli. Several of the enzymes are inhibited by serine (Bridgers, 1965), and the enzyme activity in the pre- and postnatal period shows the highest activity in the late foetal and perinatal period, a profile that closely mimics that of serine hydroxymethyl transferase (Snell, 1980). It is therefore generally agreed that this pathway is preferentially used for the synthesis of serine and glycine from glucose intermediates.

A number of observations exists on the two enzymes that are directly involved in the D-glycerate metabolism - namely D-glycerate dehydrogenase and D-glycerate kinase.

D-glycerate dehydrogenase is a dimer with identical subunits of 36000 daltons (Kitagawa *et al.*, 1975 B). Both NAD and NADP can act as co-enzyme but the activity is highest with NAD (Rosenblum *et al.*, 1971). The apparent K_m's for D-glycerate and hydroxypyruvate vary with the ionic composition of the milieu. With a sodium chloride concentration of 50 mmol/l, the K_m for D-glycerate is 500 μmol/l and the K_m for hydroxypyruvate is 44 μmol/l (Coderch, 1979). Under normal physiological conditions the equilibrium of this reaction is shifted strongly towards D-glycerate (OH-pyruvate x NADH / D-glycerate x NAD = 10^{-13}) (Dawkins and Dickens, 1965, Guynn, 1982). A number of metabolites are known to inhibit the enzyme, for example hydroxypyruvate (K_i = 80 μmol/l). In addition, inhibition of the enzyme has been demonstrated by pyruvate, 3-phosphohydroxypyruvate, fructose-1.6-diphosphate, 3-phosphoglycerate, 2.3-di-phosphoglycerate, 2-phosphoglycerate and a number of nucleotides (Sugimoto *et al.*, 1972).

In the rat, *D-glycerate kinase* has been investigated in detail in recent years. Both the mitochondrial and the cytosolic enzymes have molecular weights of about 51.000 daltons (Kitagawa *et al.*, 1979). The two enzymes have been shown to be identical in their kinetic, physical, electrochemical, chromatographic and immunochemical properties. The difference is that only the mitochondrial enzyme reacts to gluconeogenetic stimuli. Coenzyme for the enzyme is ATP (Ichihare and Greenberg, 1957). Interspecific variation is substantial. In human liver the activity is very low (Heinz *et al.*, 1968). Similarly, pig and guineapig liver have low activities, while high activities have been demonstrated in rabbit and rat tissues (Heinz, 1972, Sestoft *et al.*, 1972). The enzyme in human liver has been further investigated, and the data obtained suggested that the low activity is caused by a very high K_m value towards the D-glycerate and inhibition of the enzyme by ADP (Thieden *et al.*, 1972). In pig liver perfusion with 3 mmol/l glycerate did not cause any production of pyruvate or lactate, indicating that D-glycerate is not converted to 2-phosphoglycerate *in vivo* (Sestoft *et al.*, 1972).

5

2.1.2   The position of D-glyceric acid in the fructose degradation

Fructose is degraded mainly in the liver, the kidney, and the small intestine (Van den Berghe, 1975). Quantitatively the most important degradation pathway is via phosphorylation to fructose-1-phosphate, catalysed by ketohexokinase, followed by splitting into D-glyceraldehyde and dihydroxyacetonephosphate, catalysed by aldolase (Heinz et al., 1968),(Fig. 1). The metabolism of D-glyceraldehyde has been discussed extensively, and this point in the metabolic degradation of fructose has been called the "glyceraldehyde crossroad" (Sillero et al., 1969). As will be seen (Fig. 1) D-glyceraldehyde has 3 possible pathways for its further degradation:

A. Reduction via one of two alcohol dehydrogenases followed by phosphorylation to glycerol-1-phosphate, which is then oxidized to dihydroxyacetonephosphate.

B. Direct phosphorylation to 3-phosphoglyceraldehyde, catalysed by triokinase.

C. Oxidation to D-glycerate, catalysed by aldehyde dehydrogenase, followed by phosphorylation to 2-phosphoglycerate. However the last step in this pathway seems not to operate in humans.

A number of observations suggest that B, above, is the most prominent of these pathways. Sillero et al., (1969) have thus demonstrated that the K_m of triokinase towards D-glyceraldehyde is substantially lower than the K_m towards the two other possible enzymes and its V_{max} is relatively high. Furthermore, a number of experiments have been performed on laboratory animals, with the administration of double labelled fructose followed by determination of labelling of liver glycogen. These experiments also indicated that D-glyceraldehyde in vivo is phosphorylated via the triokinase reaction (Hue and Hers, 1972). Nevertheless, Katterman et al., (1961) have demonstrated substantial amounts of glycerate in liver tissue after intraperitoneal fructose injection and fructose infusion via the vena portae in rats. Likewise, Sestoft et al., (1972) have demonstrated substantial concentrations of glycerate in efflux media from perfused pig liver, after infusion of both fructose and D-glyceraldehyde. Both observations seem to indicate the conversion of D-glyceraldehyde to D-glycerate in vivo. The phenomenon, however, could be due to saturation of the triokinase activity by overloading with fructose. Furthermore, the demonstration of an accumulation does not clarify much about the flux through the pathway. The observations probably reflect the low in vivo activity of the D-glycerate kinase. In this connection it seems relevant that neither the mitochondrial nor the cytoplasmatic D-glycerate kinase is induced by fructose administration (Kitagawa et al., 1979). Conversion of the D-glycerate to hydroxypyruvate (catalysed by D-glycerate dehydrogenase) is probably very low due to the fact that the D-glycerate dehydrogenase reaction is normally shifted strongly towards D-glycerate (Dawkins and Dickens, 1965).

In conclusion it can be said that in man, the D-glyceraldehyde formed in the degradation of fructose is normally metabolised via phosphorylation to 3-phosphoglyceraldehyde, catalysed by triokinase. In the event of overloading,

6

a smaller part can be transformed to D-glycerate which is not phosphorylated and therefore accumulates. In man and other species with low *in vivo* D-glycerate kinase activity, D-glycerate seems to be an end metabolite (Heinz *et al.*, 1968).

2.2 THE HYPERGLYCERIC ACIDEMIAS

Apart from the patient with hyper-D-glyceric acidemia and hyperglycinemia described in section 4, a number of different clinical and biochemical pictures have been described in which hyperglyceric acidemia occurs.

2.2.1 L-glyceric acidemia

In 1968 Williams and Smith described four patients, (three of which were siblings) who all excreted oxalate stones in the urine as a dominant clinical symptom. Between these attacks, the patients were healthy. Initially the patients were suspected of suffering from primary oxaluria (type I), but further investigations showed that they excreted greatly elevated amounts of L-glyceric acid and oxalic acid in urine, but not increased amounts of glycolic acid as in primary oxaluria (type I). Further investigations demonstrated diminished D-glycerate dehydrogenase activity in leucocytes from one of the patients. The authors thought that the L-glyceric acid excretion was caused by this deficiency (Williams and Smith, 1968 A and B). This hypothesis was based on the assumption that the flux through pathway II was to the right (Fig. 1), causing accumulation of hydroxypyruvic acid, which, catalysed by lactate dehydrogenase, was converted to L-glyceric acid. No other explanation of the L-glyceric aciduria has been presented to date. However an accumulation of hydroxypyruvic acid has never been verified and oral L-serine loading tests (10 g/day) did not lead to increased urinary excretion of L-glyceric acid, which would be expected with the proposed metabolic derangement.

The hyperoxaluria was not explained satisfactorily either. In the first description of the patients, the authors tried to demonstrate a possible precursor-product relationship between oxalic acid and hydroxypyruvic acid, by a number of tracer studies. These indicated that there was no metabolic interconversion between precursors of oxalate and glycerate in the patient. In a later publication (Williams and Smith, 1971), the authors suggested that hydroxypyruvic acid (like pyruvate), stimulates the oxidation of glycolate to oxalate. The authors therefore suggested that the effect could be caused by a shift in the NAD-NADH ratio caused by hydroxypyruvic acid which should stimulate the oxidation of glycolate. Later publications from Richardson and co-workers have, however, questioned this hypothesis (Liao and Richardson, 1978). Instead, these workers found indications for the conversion of hydroxypyruvate to oxalate both by auto-oxidation and enzyme-catalyzed oxidation (Liao and Richardson, 1978; Raghavan and Richardson, 1983). To date, this group suggests that the oxalate excretion in these patients is due to

7

nonmetabolised hydroxypyruvate being accumulated in tissue and converted to oxalate.

It must thus be concluded that while the excretion pattern has been characterised in detail, the basic metabolic derangement is still not fully understood and needs further investigations.

2.2.2   D-glyceric acidemia with chronic acidosis

In 1976 another group of workers (Wadman *et al.*, 1976) described a boy who developed tachypnoe, tachycardia and severe metabolic acidosis from the age of 13 days. Further biochemical investigations demonstrated an isolated accumulation of D-glyceric acid in blood and urine.

Measurements of amino acids in blood and urine initially showed a moderate, generalized amino aciduria, but later normal values were found. The child responded favourably to treatment with bicarbonate and a low protein diet. On this treatment the child became clinically normal with a satisfactory development up to the age of 4 1/2 months, at which time the group lost contact with the patient.

At the age of 16 months the child was admitted to another hospital for a short period. Clinical examination gave the impression that the child was moderately mentally retarded, but his parents would not allow any further examinations or follow up. The only investigations aimed at elucidating the etiology of the patient's hyper-D-glyceric acidemia were a number of *in vivo* loading tests. It was shown that fructose loading did not increase the D-glyceric acid excretion or aggravate the acidosis. On two occasions serine loading increased the D-glyceric acid accumulation, however. It was demonstrated that the increase in D-glyceric acid excretion in the first 6 hours after loading corresponded to 14% of the administered serine.

On the basis of these results Wadman and co-workers (Wadman *et al.*, 1976) have considered the basic defect. It seems evident from the results of the serine loading test on this patient that pathway II is intact from serine to D-glyceric acid, with a flux towards the right (Fig. 1). The D-glycerate dehydrogenase must therefore be assumed to be normal in this child. The D-glyceric acid accumulation could, theoretically, be caused by deficiency of D-glycerate kinase. However, the *in vivo* D-glycerate kinase activity in man is so low, that a strong flux towards the right in pathway II might cause hyper-D-glyceric acidemia, as also pointed out by the authors. As an alternative hypothesis the authors suggested a defect in serine metabolism, which would cause such a flux. However, as explained later, with our present knowledge of serine metabolism it is difficult to suggest an enzyme defect which would shunt a large part of the administered serine into pathway II. The fact that fructose loading did not give increased D-glyceric acid excretion seems to suggest that fructose in the patient was mainly metabolized via D-glyceraldehyde and 3-phosphoglyceraldehyde,

8

i.e. via the normal pathway.

It can therefore be concluded that the basic defect is unknown and, due to the complicated biochemical position of D-glyceric acid, it seems impossible at present to formulate a hypothesis that can explain the loading tests.

2.2.3   D-glyceric acidemia with cerebral dysfunction

The Dutch group which described the previous patient has also examined a mentally retarded girl with excretion of D-glyceric acid (Duran *et al.*, 1988). Clinically this patient was hypotonic from birth, had slow motor development and had seizures from the age of one year. In addition to a prominent peak for D-glyceric acid, the organic acid profile showed multiple peaks due to valproate medication. No other organic acids were elevated and amino acids were normal. The D-glyceric acid excretion increased substantially after fructose and dihydroxyacetone loading, but not after serine loading. Enzyme studies were performed only on erytrocytes, where various glycolytic enzymes were measured. Apart from a slightly diminished glyceraldehyd-3-phosphate dehydrogenase these enzyme measurements gave normal results (including normal triokinase).

The basic defect in this child is unknown, but the loading data clearly indicate a metabolic derangement different from the previously described patient. A possible explanation could be a defect somewhere in the fructose degradation, shunting glyceraldehyde down into the "blind alley" of D-glyceric acid.

2.2.4   Other cases with excretion of D-glyceric acid

Grandgeorge (thesis, Grenoble, 1979) has described another child with hyper-D-glyceric acidemia. The child was normal at birth, but at 3 weeks of age developed progressive neurological symptoms in the form of hypotonia, epistotonus and myoclonias and died 4 1/2 months old. Glycine concentrations in blood and urine were marginally elevated, cerebrospinal fluid glycine concentrations were not measured. No attempts to explain the etiology of the hyper-D-glyceric acidemia were made. However, a post mortem examination of the central nervous system was performed. Microspongiosis diffusa was demonstrated and a slight demyelination. These changes seem similar to the changes that have been described in nonketotic hyperglycinemia (Agamanolis *et al.*, 1982). Due to the limited amount of data available, it is at present difficult to classify this patient, but he seems strikingly similar to the Dutch girl described above.

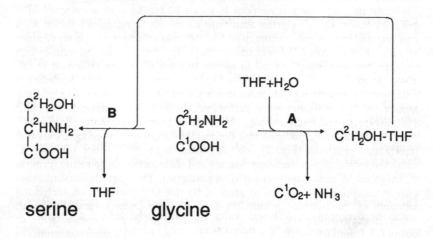

Fig. 2.   The relationship between the serine hydroxymethyl transferase-catalyzed process (B) and the glycine cleavage-catalyzed process (A). The two carbon atoms of glycine are marked C^1 and C^2

3. THE HYPERGLYCINEMIAS

3.1 THE NORMAL METABOLISM OF GLYCINE

Glycine is present in all tissues and constitutes as much as 25% of collagen and elastine. Normal adults consume about 3-5 g per day, (Rosenberg and Scriver, 1980). In humans, the glycine pool is about 80 mg/kg with a turnover of 1 g/kg/24 hours. Of ^{15}N-glycine administered to rats in nitrogen balance 40% was excreted unchanged in urine, whereas 45% was retained in the body (Ratner *et al.*, 1940). After administration of ^{14}C-glycine, the protein-bound radioactivity was mainly found in serine and not in glycine (Winnick *et al.*, 1948). It was therefore initially thought that the most prominent degradation pathway for glycine was via conversion to serine. In the following years a number of tracer studies were performed, both in intact animals (Sakami, 1948,1949; Arnstein and Neuberg, 1953), and in liver homogenates (Sato *et al.*, 1969 A). These studies indicate that the metabolism of glycine proceeds via two interrelated processes (Fig. 2), viz: degradation to the C_1-pool (process A, catalysed by the glycine cleavage system) and transformation to serine (process B, catalysed by serine hydroxymethyl transferase). The interrelationship exists only in conditions with excess of glycine. By the administration of decreasing amounts of ^{14}C-2-glycine (from 2% to 0.1% of the daily intake) to rats, Arnstein and Neuberg (1953) found that the labelling of the 3-carbon-atom of serine fell from 60% of the specific activity of the glycine's 2-carbon atom, to about 10%. This indicates that at low glycine loads, the C_1-units forming the 3-carbon atom of the serine molecules synthesized does not preferentially come from reaction A, but also from the endogeneous (and therefore unlabelled) C_1-pool.

The two enzyme systems involved in reactions A and B will be treated separately before other relevant metabolic pathways are described

11

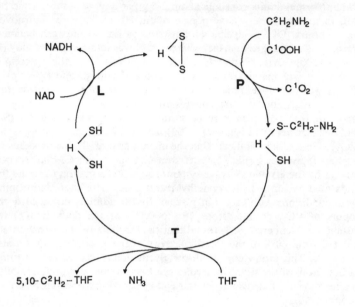

Fig. 3.   The reaction sequence of the glycine cleavage system. The four
protein components P-, H-, T-and L-protein are indicated and the
two carbon atoms of glycine are marked C^1 and C^2.

12

3.1.1 Serine-glycine interconversion

This process is catalysed by the enzyme serine hydroxymethyl transferase

$$\text{L-serine} + \text{THF} \rightleftarrows \text{Glycine} + 5.10\text{-}CH_2\text{-}THF + H_2O$$

It is fully reversible, but is generally considered to be shifted towards the right and, together with the glycine cleavage process, to be the most important pathway for the generation of C_1-fragments (Kikuchi, 1973). The enzyme has been purified to homogeneity from rat, rabbit, sheep, ox and monkey, and consists of two isoenzymes. One is located in the cytoplasm and the other in the mitochondrial matrix (Ogawa and Fujika, 1981). The kinetic constants have been found to be similar (K_m for serine $= 0.54$ mmol/l, K_m for glycine $= 1.5$ mmol/l) for the two isoenzymes (Nakano et al., 1968). In the serine/glycine interconversion, tetrahydrofolic acid (THF) participates as cofactor with a K_m of about 0.1 mmol/l. Serine hydroxymethyl transferase has been demonstrated in a number of organs (liver, kidney, spleen, testis, brain, heart, lungs, muscles and intestine) in higher animals and in insects, bacteria and plants (Kikuchi et al., 1980).

Since serine hydroxymethyl transferase catalyses a process which generates C_1-fragments, it is not surprising that the C_1-homeostasis seems to have a regulatory effect on this enzyme. It has been shown that serine hydroxymethyl transferase from monkey liver is inhibited by methylated THF-derivatives (5-CH_2-THF and 5-CHO-THF) (Ramesh and Rao, 1980). In addition, evidence has been obtained from bacterial systems that both methionine and S-adenosylmethionine act as co-repressors on serine hydroxymethyl transferase synthesis (Meedel and Pizer, 1974; Greene and Radovich, 1975).

3.1.2 The glycine cleavage system

At present, this enzyme system is considered to catalyse the quantitatively most important degradation route for glycine. The system is rather complicated and resembles in many ways the oxidative decarboxylation systems that degrade pyruvic acid and 2-ketoglutaric acid. It is a multienzyme system involving several metabolic steps and several co-enzymes (Fig. 3).

The enzyme system has been investigated extensively by Kikuchi and co-workers, and they have named the four enzyme components involved viz: P, H, T, and L-proteins (Kikuchi and Higara, 1982)

P-protein is the glycine decarboxylase (Hiraga and Kikuchi, 1980 A), and contains two pyridoxal phosphate groups. Its activity can be measured both as $^{14}CO_2$ production from ^{14}C-1-glycine and as $^{14}CO_2$ exchange between NaH$^{14}CO_3$ and glycine in the reaction mixture. The P-protein alone can catalyse both these reactions although very slowly (Hiraga and Kikuchi, 1980 B). The velocity of both reactions is stimulated (up to 300 times) by addition of

13

H-protein. With highly purified P- and H-protein it has been shown, that a rather stable complex is formed during the enzyme catalysis, followed by conformational changes in the P-protein (Hiraga and Kikuchi, 1980 B).

The *H-protein* itself has a molecular weight of about 14.500 and contains one molecule of lipoic acid per molecule (Fujikawa *et al.*, 1979). It has been demonstrated that in both the decarboxylation and in the exchange reaction, H-protein can be substituted by lipoic acid (Hiraga and Kikuchi, 1980 A). In addition, it has been demonstrated that the H-protein is a carrier for the C_2-carbon-atom of glycine after decarboxylation. The amino methyl fragment is attached to one of the S atoms of the oxidized lipoic acid groups (Fig. 3). The H-protein therefore has three functions in the decarboxylation, first as modulator of the P-protein, then as electron acceptor and finally as carrier for the amino methyl group after glycine decarboxylation (Hiraga and Kikuchi, 1980 B).

Of the remaining two components of the glycine cleavage system, the *T-protein* is the enzyme which catalyses the transfer of the H-protein bound amino methyl group to a THF, followed by release of NH_3 (Okamura-Ikeda *et al.*, 1982). In this process THF participates as a necessary cofactor.

The last component in the glycine cleavage system is the L-protein. *L-protein* is a lipoyl dehydrogenase which catalyses the reoxidation of H-protein with NAD as cofactor. It has not been characterized in higher animals. Therefore it is not known whether the glycine cleavage system has its own specific lipoyl dehydrogenase, or if L-protein is identical to the lipoyl dehydrogenase participating in the dehydrogenation of 2-oxo acids.

The overall reaction for the total glycine cleavage system is thus:

$$GLYCINE + THF + NAD \rightleftarrows 5.10\text{-}CH_2\text{-}THF + CO_2 + NH_3 + NADH + H^+$$

This process is fully reversible. From left to right it is a glycine cleavage, whereas from right to left it is a glycine synthesis.

In rat liver, the K_m towards glycine is around 1 mmol/l when glycine cleavage activity is measured (Motokawa and Kikuchi, 1974), whereas values from 2.7 to 7 mmol/l have been found when CO_2 exchange was measured (Hayasaka *et al.*, 1980, Hayasaka and Tada, 1983). With intact mitochondria, K_m's have been measured in the range 3-10 mmol/l (Sato *et al.*, 1969 B; Kølvraa, 1979; Hampton *et al.*, 1983).

With reference to the intracellular localisation of the glycine cleavage system, it has been demonstrated that the enzyme system is exclusively intramitochondrial and bound as a complex to the inner membrane (Motokawa and Kikuchi, 1971). The enzyme system is thus localised in the same compartment as the mitochondrial serine hydroxymethyl transferase, but is not solubilized as easily (Motokawa and Kikuchi, 1971). Studies on the organ distribution of the glycine

14

cleavage system have demonstrated highest activity in liver tissue and lower activity in kidney, central nervous system and testis. All other organs have no detectable activity (Yoshida and Kikuchi, 1972). Pronounced differences exist between species (Yoshida and Kikuchi, 1972). The glycine cleavage activity in human liver tissue is of the same magnitude as found in rats, which is the animal that has been investigated in most detail (de Groot et al., 1970). The role of the glycine cleavage system in the central nervous system will be treated in detail in the section describing the role of glycine as a neurotransmitter.

Very little is known about the regulation of the glycine cleavage system. Hampton et al.,(1983, 1984) have investigated the effect of mitochondrial reduction. These workers found that increasing intramitochondrial NADH and NADPH concentrations inhibited the glycine cleavage system, both in isolated mitochondria and in perfused livers. The inhibitory effect of NADH is not surprising, since this compound is a cofactor of the reaction. Why NADPH also affects the reaction is less evident and at present not convincingly explained.

3.1.3   The relationship between the metabolism of glycine and serine

A number of observations indicate that serine is normally degraded via the serine hydroxymethyl transferase-catalysed reaction to glycine and that the degradation of glycine mainly occurs via the glycine cleavage system.

In addition to the serine hydroxymethyl transferase catalysed pathway, serine can be degraded via conversion to pyruvate, catalysed by serine hydratase and via conversion to hydroxypyruvic acid, catalysed by serine pyruvate aminotransferase (Fig. 1). It is difficult to compare the relative activities of these three enzymes in liver tissue since they are located in different cellular compartments (Snell, 1975, Ogawa and Fujika, 1981). It would seem, however, that liver tissue from various animals generally contains the highest activity of serine hydroxymethyl transferase followed by serine hydratase and the lowest activity of serine pyruvate aminotransferase (Snell, 1975, Yoshida and Kikuchi, 1973), indicating a preferential degradation of serine via glycine. In this context, it is of relevance that Snell (1986) was unable to demonstrate serine hydratase in human liver. Tracer studies with administration of ^{14}C-3-serine on intact animals (Kretchmar and Price, 1969; Elwyn, 1957) also indicated transformation to glycine to be the most important degradation pathway for serine. A detailed review of serine metabolism has resently been published by Snell (1984).

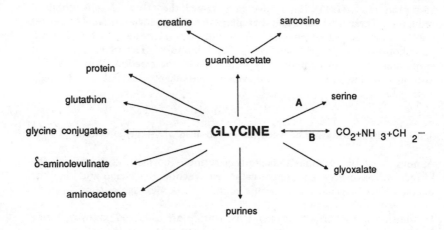

Fig. 4.   The normal metabolism of glycine. A: serine hydroxymethyl transferase; B: the glycine cleavage system.

16

Glycine is the amino acid which has the greatest number of possible metabolic pathways (Fig. 4). Apart from conversion to serine, only two of these pathways are catabolic, namely glycine cleavage and transamination to glyoxylate, catalysed by amino acid oxidase (Dixon and Kleppe, 1965; Ratner et al., 1944). Since both enzymes are present in kidney tissue, this organ has been used in quantitative degradation studies. Such studies have shown that the glycine oxidation in kidney homogenate has a cofactor requirement corresponding to a glycine cleavage reaction (Rowsell et al., 1982). Furthermore, it has been demonstrated that glyoxylate, which is the product of the amino acid oxidase reaction, does not inhibit this glycine oxidation (Rowsell et al., 1982, Yoshida and Kikuchi, 1973). These findings clearly suggest that even in kidney tissue, where amino acid oxidase activity is known to be very high, degradation via glycine cleavage is predominant.

The other reactions shown in Fig. 4 are all synthetic pathways. As such, most of them are probably under synthetic control and therefore an increase in flux into these pathways caused by accumulation of glycine, will probably be very modest. An exception is glycine conjugation, which might be of importance in patients with certain types of hyperglycinemia. This glycine conjugation mechanism is described below.

3.2   THE BIOLOGICAL ROLE OF GLYCINE

In the preceding section the degradation of glycine has been described. In this connection, the role of glycine as C_1-donor and as serine-precursor has also been described. Further, glycine also participates in a number of synthetic processes as depicted in Fig. 4. In addition, a substantial amount of evidence collected during recent years indicates that glycine plays a role as neuro-transmitter in the central nervous system. Two of these functions are important for understanding the pathogenesis in various types of hyperglycinemia. These are glycine conjugation of toxic substances and the role of glycine in the central nervous system, and they are described here.

3.2.1   Glycine conjugation of toxic substances

It is generally agreed that detoxification by conjugation has been developed in animals to facilitate the removal of various plant acids which the animals are not able to degrade. Other types of molecules such as drugs (Forman et al., 1971) and accumulated endogeneous metabolites (Gregersen, 1985) are also conjugated. Conjugation to sugars, amino acids and certain other compounds, such as carnitine, occur. A number of amino acids (glycine, glutamine, taurine, arginine, asparagine, histidine, ornithine, cysteine, lysine and serine) are substrates for conjugation in different species, but glycine conjugation seems generally to be most common and biologically most important (James et al., 1972, Webster et al., 1976). The enzyme that catalyses the glycine conjugation of accumulated endogeneous metabolites is called benzoyl-CoA:glycine

N-acyltransferase, since available data indicate that the natural substrates are benzoyl-CoA and glycine and the natural product is hippuric acid. The enzyme has been known since the beginning of the fifties, when Schachter and Taggart (1953) demonstrated the ability of acetone-dried ox liver mitochondrial powder to synthesize hippuric acid. They originally called the enzyme glycine-N-acylase.

The enzyme, which is present in large amounts in liver mitochondria (Gatley and Sherratt, 1977; Kølvraa and Gregersen, 1986) catalyses the formation of acylglycine from acyl-CoA and glycine, under liberation of CoA:

$$\text{Acyl-CoA + Glycine} \rightarrow \text{Acylglycine + CoA}$$

The formation of the peptide bond is an energy-dependent process. The energy needed is delivered by the CoA-ester of the acyl substrate, a CoA ester which is synthetised in an ATP-dependent process *in vivo* (Schachter and Taggart, 1953).

The significance of the observation that this enzyme also conjugates aliphatic acids (Schachter & Taggart, 1953) remained unappreciated until the development of gas chromatographic/mass spectrometric techniques in the 1960's. Researchers were then able to demonstrate the existence of a number of i.e.o.m. in the degradation pathways of amino acids (Tanaka *et al.*, 1966, Oberholzer *et al.*, 1967, Hommes *et al.*, 1968, Keating *et al.*, 1972) and later of fatty acids (Gregersen *et al.*, 1976, Mantagos *et al.*, 1979, Truscott *et al.*, 1979), all of which had the excretion in urine of various low molecular weight organic acids as a dominant feature. These patients excreted a number of glycine conjugates of short, aliphatic fatty acids such as propionylglycine, isobutyrylglycine, butyrylglycine, isovalerylglycine, 2-methylbutyrylglycine, hexanoylglycine, octanoylglycine, suberylglycine and succinylglycine (Gregersen, 1985).

Prompted by these findings, the substrate-specificity and the kinetic constants of the enzyme towards the various substrates were investigated. The K_m for benzoyl-CoA was demonstrated to be in the range 6 - 40 μmol/l, depending on the species (Lau *et al.*, 1977; Webster *et al.*, 1976). When using benzoyl-CoA as cosubstrate, the K_m for glycine was found to be between 3 - 20 mmol/l. Detailed enzyme kinetic studies indicated a sequential reaction mechanism (Nandi *et al.*, 1979).

The kinetic constants towards different aliphatic acyl-CoA's have also been investigated on liver tissue from several species including man (Bartlett and Gompertz, 1974; Webster *et al.*, 1976; Kølvraa and Gregersen, 1986; Gregersen *et al.*, 1986). Working on human liver, Gregersen and coworkers (Gregersen *et al.*, 1986) found K_m values for all acyl-CoA's to range from 300 - 5000 μmol/l. There seems to be no clear correlation between affinity and length or branching of the carbon chain.

When acyl-CoA's were co-substrate, K_m values towards glycine of over 1000 mmol/l were found, with human enzyme (Gregersen *et al.*, 1986).

Only a few investigators have studied the possible regulation of glycine-N-acylase. The question as to whether glycine-N-acylase can be induced has been investigated by James and Bendt (1978) by administering benzoic acid both orally and intraperitonally to rats and then measuring the activity of glycine-N-acylase in liver tissue. Unfortunately they used phenylacetyl-CoA as substrate in the enzyme assay, thereby risking false conclusions, as rats have different enzymes which catalyse the glycine conjugation of benzoyl-CoA and phenylacetyl-CoA (Nandi *et al.*, 1979). With this reservation in mind, the work indicates that neither benzoic acid administration nor administration of salicylic acid (natural substrate for phenylacetyl-CoA:glycine N-acyltransferase) gave measurable induction of the enzyme. For man, the high K_m values for aliphatic acyl-CoA's and the corresponding high K_m values for glycine (Gregersen *et al.*, 1986) suggest that glycine conjugation of aliphatic acids can be stimulated by increasing intramitochondrial concentrations of substrates. Some support for this hypothesis with regards to acyl-CoA's is shown by the fact that aliphatic acylglycines in man are almost exclusively seen in connection with i.e.o.m., i.e. in situations where the acyl-CoA's must be assumed to accumulate in liver tissue. Regarding glycine, support for this hypothesis is lent by the fact that in patients with isovaleryl-CoA dehydrogenase deficiency, the excretion of isovalerylglycine can be increased substantially during attacks by treatment with glycine (Krieger and Tanaka, 1976).

3.2.2   The role of glycine as neuro-transmitter

It is generally agreed that the following criteria have to be met before a substance can be considered to be a neuro-transmitter:

A.   The substance has to be unevenly distributed in the central nervous system, a distribution which is difficult to explain by more general metabolic functions. It is reasonable to assume that the highest concentration is in areas where other available data suggest that the neuro-physiological function is exerted.

B.   The substance is liberated when the neurones are stimulated by depolarisation.

C.   Application of the substance to the area of the synapse causes effects which are similar to those caused by natural neuro-transmitters.

D.   The existence of an effective system for removal of the substance from the effector-area immediately after the effect has occurred.

Glycine fulfills all these criteria. Glycine was originally suggested as a neuro-transmitter (Aprison and Werman, 1965) after it had been demonstrated that a pronounced rostrocaudal gradient for glycine existed in the central nervous system. The concentration in the medulla spinalis is 3-5 times higher than the concentration in the cerebrum (Davis & Johnston, 1973, 1974; Berger *et al.*, 1977; Kontro *et al.*, 1980). The detailed distribution of glycine within the medulla spinalis has also been investigated in several species. It has been shown that the glycine concentration is unexpectedly high in the anterior horns and the white substance localized there (Miyata and Otsuka, 1975; Berger *et al.*, 1977; Patric *et al.*, 1983). As pointed out by several authors, this distribution is very specific for glycine (Davis and Johnston, 1973) and is difficult to associate with other metabolic functions. Glycine thus meets criterion A.

In intact medulla spinalis preparations, in slices from the medulla spinalis and also in purified synaptosomes, depolarisation-mediated release of ^{14}C-glycine occurs when the preparations have been pre-incubated with this compound (Roberts and Mitchell, 1972; Ehinger and Lindberg-Bauer, 1976; Cutler *et al.*, 1972; Bradford *et al.*, 1973). Glycine thus meets criterion B.

Glycine applied to medulla spinalis preparations hyperpolarises spinal, motory neurons and lowers the frequency of impulses in a manner similar to that found by natural inhibitory transmitter substances (Werman *et al.*, 1968; Curtis *et al.*, 1968 A and B). Several observations indicate that this effect is achieved by the binding of glycine to a specific receptor postsynaptically, which results in the opening of a group of chloride channels (Gold and Martin, 1983 and 1984). The interest in the hyperpolarising effect of glycine was stimulated when it was demonstrated that this effect could be removed by small doses of strychnine. Binding studies have documented that glycine and strychnine compete on the same postsynaptic receptor although probably on two different sites (Young and Schneider, 1973; Snyder, 1975). In accordance with this finding it has been demonstrated that the distribution of strychnine-binding sites in the central nervous system corresponds closely to both the distribution of endogeneous glycine and to that of the high-affinity glycine-uptake system (Young and Schneider, 1973; Johnson and Iversen, 1971). Glycine thus meets criterion C.

The fourth criterion for neuro-transmitter function, the existence of a mechanism for effective removal from the synapse-cleft, is also fulfilled. Two uptake systems, a high affinity system and a low affinity system, which transfer glycine into the cells, have been demonstrated both in slices and homogenates from various areas of the central nervous system from various animals. In cortex, cerebellum and midbrain, a low affinity system with K_m-values for glycine ranging from 200-300 μmol/l dominates (Johnston and Iversen, 1971; Davidoff and Adair, 1976), while in the lower part of the central nervous system, a high affinity uptake system dominates with K_m about 20 μmol/l (Davidoff and Adair, 1975; Davidoff and Adair, 1976; Johnston and Iversen, 1971; Balcar and Johnston, 1973). The location of the high affinity uptake system in medulla spinalis has been identified in the synaptosomal fraction (Balcar and Johnston, 1973; Johnston and Iversen, 1971; Logan and Schneider, 1972; Hökfelt and Ljungdahl, 1971). The distribution of the high affinity uptake system therefore closely mimics firstly the distribution of endogeneous glycine, secondly the distribution of glycine binding sites and thirdly the distribution of areas where glycine exerts neuro-physiological effects.

The substrate specificity of the high affinity uptake system differs from that of the low affinity uptake system. While the low affinity uptake system transports a number of other amino acids (Johnston and Iversen, 1971) and seems to correspond to the ASC-system described by Christensen (1975), the high affinity uptake system is highly specific for glycine (Johnston and Iversen, 1971; Blacar and Johnston, 1973; Davidoff and Adair, 1976). It is therefore generally agreed that while the low affinity system is a general system for the central nervous system and serves more general metabolic functions, the high affinity system is located exclusively in the synapse-cleft. This is where glycine is liberated as a neuro-transmitter and where specific and fast removal is needed after the neuro-physiological effect has occured.

Available data indicate that the extracellular fluid of the central nervous system including that in the synaptic area, is in open connection with the cerebrospinal fluid (Bito et al., 1966) and it is not surprising therefore that glycine is present in extremely low concentrations in the cerebrospinal fluid. The plasma:cerebrospinal fluid ratio for glycine is 20-40:1, while for most other amino acids it is below 10:1 (Perry et al., 1975). Two systems participate in maintaining this pronounced concentration gradient between blood and cerebrospinal fluid. These are the uptake systems described earlier and a very effective blood-brain barrier for glycine. It has been shown that glycine uptake during the passage of radioactive glycine through the vascular system of the central nervous system is practically zero. This is contrary to most other amino acids (Pollay, 1975; Oldendorf, 1971), which equilibrate with the cerebral amino acid pool. Furthermore, a transport system may exist which removes glycine from the cerebrospinal fluid directly into the bloodstream, possibly via the plexus chorioideus (Murray and Cutler, 1970; Dudzinski and Cutler, 1974).

Since a very efficient blood-brain barrier for glycine exists, it can be assumed that the glycine pool of the central nervous system is separated from the glycine pool of the rest of the body. This makes the cerebral synthesis and degradation of glycine very important. Glycine synthesis in the central nervous system has been investigated by Shank and co-workers in a number of tracer studies (Shank and Aprison, 1970; Shank et al., 1973). They indicated that the greater part of free glycine in the brain is synthesized from serine, probably with glucose and glycolytic intermediates as precursors. In accordance with this, it appears that the distribution of serine hydroxymethyl transferase in the central nervous system corresponds reasonably well with the distribution of endogeneous glycine (Daly and Aprison, 1974; Davis and Johnston, 1973). In addition, Bridgers (1965) demonstrated that serine synthesis from glycolytic intermediates seems to occur preferentially via the phosphorylated pathway, analogous to the system seen in liver.

Catabolism of glycine in the central nervous system is considered to occur

21

predominantly via the glycine cleavage system. As previously mentioned this system has been demonstrated to be active in the central nervous system. Initially, the importance of the glycine cleavage system was underestimated, since the distribution of enzyme activity did not correspond to that of the glycine concentrations (Uhr, 1973; Bruin *et al.*, 1973). Evaluations of the distribution of the glycine cleavage system in the central nervous system are hampered, however, by the existence of an endogeneous inhibitor (Daly *et al.*, 1976). The distribution of this inhibitor shows a rostrocaudal gradient analogous to the endogeneous glycine concentration and can therefore very well mask a latent activity, especially in the medulla spinalis. Only very little is known about this inhibitor apart from it being of high molecular weight, thermolabile, and that an increase in NAD-concentration partly abolishes its effect (Daly *et al.*, 1976). Its biological role is still not clear.

The "cycle" of the glycine in the central nervous system can be summarized as follows: 1. Synthesis from glucose via serine in the cytosol of the neurones; 2. Transport to the presynaptic membranes possibly in the axonal transport vesicles (Price and McAdoo, 1981); 3. Liberation in the synapse-clefts by a stimulus of depolarization; 4: High affinity uptake into the cells using the high affinity uptake system, followed either by re-use in the transmitter pool or by degradation via the glycine cleavage system.

3.3   THE HYPERGLYCINEMIA SYNDROMES

3.3.1   Historic aspects

In 1961, Childs and Nyhan (Childs *et al.*, 1961; Nyhan *et al.*, 1961) described a 3 year-old boy with a syndrome characterized by periods of ketoacidosis, vomiting and lethargy. During attacks, laboratory investigations demonstrated both leucocytopenia and thrombocytopenia. Investigations of amino acids in blood and urine showed elevated concentrations of a number of amino acids, among which glycine dominated. In addition, it was demonstrated that administration of five amino acids, namely isoleucine, leucine, valine, methionine and threonine deteriorated the clinical condition. This syndrome was named iodopatic hyperglycinemia.

In the following years several patients with this syndrome were described (Tada *et al.*, 1963; Cochrane *et al.*, 1963; Nyhan *et al.*, 1963), but cases also appeared which clearly deviated from the picture mentioned (Mabry and Karam, 1963; Schreier and Müller, 1964; Gerritsen *et al.*, 1965). These children exhibited a different clinical picture, namely hypotonia, lethargy, lack of reflexes and myoclonias in the neonatal period; they often died very young. Episodes of ketoacidosis, vomiting and leuco- or thrombocytopenia did not occure. On examination of the amino acids isolated hyperglycinemia and hyperglycinuria were present and deterioration of the clinical condition was demonstrated following administration of serine, but not after administration of leucine

22

(Gerritsen *et al.*, 1965). Based on these findings Rampini *et al.* (1967), suggested subdividing the syndrome iodopatic hyperglycinemia into two distinct entities: ketotic hyperglycinemia (the original iodopatic hyperglycinemia) and nonketotic hyperglycinemia.

3.3.2 "Ketotic" hyperglycinemia

In the years following this discovery a number of groups worked intensively on the elucidation of the causal defect in the syndrome "ketotic hyperglycinemia". To begin with, most researchers concentrated on glycine metabolism in these patients and a number of observations were presented.

Nyhan and Childs (1964) investigated the turnover and pool size of glycine on the original patient. As would be expected they demonstrated a somewhat greater glycine pool in the patient, but the pool turnover was normal, which means that when the results are expressed in grams glycine, the turnover in the patient was almost twice that found in controls. The only other amino acid that was labelled when giving radioactive glycine was serine. This labelling was demonstrated to be slightly less in the patient than in controls. Based on these findings, a defect in glycine-serine conversion was suggested (Nyhan and Childs, 1964), a hypothesis which was hampered by the fact that the authors did not try to correct the degree of labelling of serine for the differences in glycine pool size between patient and control.

A number of groups studied the degradation of glycine via transamination to glyoxylate and further to oxalate. This line of research was intensified when Gerritsen *et al.* (1965), in their first publication on the syndrome nonketotic hyperglycinemia demonstrated "hypo-oxaluria". Rampini *et al.*, (1967), however, performed detailed measurements on glyoxylate and oxalate in urine from patients with both the "ketotic" and the nonketotic types of hyperglycinemia and concluded that no abnormalities in oxalate metabolism seemed to exist in either.

3.3.2.1 Methylmalonic acidemia

A breakthrough came from an entirely different line of research and was prompted by the fact that administration of the branched-chain amino acids leucine, isoleucine, and valine deteriorated the clinical condition in children with "ketotic" hyperglycinemia.

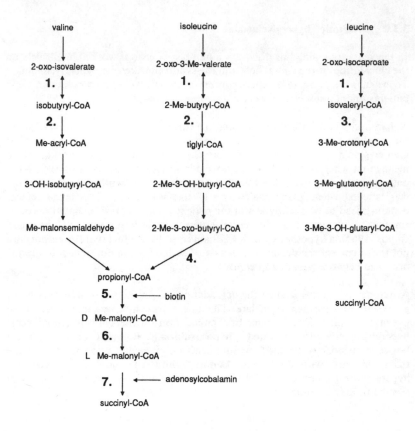

Fig 5.   The normal metabolism of branched-chain amino acids. 1.:
2-oxo-acid   decarboxylase;   2.:   branched-chain   acyl-CoA
dehydrogenase;   3.:   isovaleryl-CoA   dehydrogenase;   4.:
β-ketothiolase;   5.:   propionyl-CoA   carboxylase;   6.:
D-methylmalonyl-CoA   rasemase;   7.:   L-methylmalonyl-CoA
mutase.

In 1967 Oberholzer and et al., (1967), described excretion of methylmalonic acid in urine from two children. The children presented persistent acidosis, complicated by acute deteriorations provoked by trival infections. One of these children had hyperglycinemia on several occasions and thus fulfilled the criteria for having "ketotic" hyperglycinemia. As can be seen in Fig. 5. methylmalonyl-CoA is an intermediate in the degradation of isoleucine and valine, and a block at enzyme 6 or 7 will give rise to severe methylmalonic aciduria. During the following years, a number of patients with "ketotic" hyperglycinemia were investigated for methylmalonic acid excretion and it soon became evident that "ketotic" hyperglycinemia was biochemically heterogeneous, since it occurred both in patients with and without methylmalonic acidemia. The syndrome of methylmalonic acidemia combined with hyperglycinemia was then separated as a distinct entity and it was soon observed that methylmalonic acidemia could occur both with and without concomitant hyperglycinemia (Nyhan et al., 1972). Later it appeared that methylmalonic acidemia in itself is very heterogeneous and can be caused by a number of different biochemical defects. At present, 6 different inherited biochemical defects have been located: two in the mutase-apoenzyme and four in different positions of the vitamin B_{12}-metabolism. The B_{12} metabolite adenosylcobalamine is the prostetic group of methylmalonyl-CoA mutase (Rosenberg, 1983).

A more detailed description of the various methylmalonic acidemias, their biochemical and clinical characteristics and their treatment is outside the scope of the present review, which focuses on hyperglycinemia. It has not been possible to correlate the presence or absence of hyperglycinemia with any of the above mentioned subgroups.

3.3.2.2   Propionic acidemia

Following the demonstration of methylmalonic acidemia, "ketotic" hyperglycinemia was further subdivided when a defect in the degradation of propionic acid was demonstrated in several patients. Interest in the propionic acid metabolism in these patients stemmed from the fact that isoleucine, valine, threonine and methionine - four of the five amino acids that patients with "ketotic" hyperglycinemia did not tolerate - were common precursors for propionic acid. In addition Hommes et al. (1968), had described a child with a lethal, neonatal ketoacidosis who excreted more than 1000 times the normal amounts of propionic acid. Glycine in blood and urine was normal in this child, but the clinical picture resembled that seen in severe neonatal "ketotic" hyperglycinemia. In the years that followed, both severe accumulation of propionic acid (Gompertz et al., 1970; Ando et al., 1971 B) and diminished oxidation of propionic acid (Hsia et al., 1969; Hsia et al., 1971) were demonstrated in a number of patients. Based on these findings, propionyl CoA carboxylase deficiency (propionic acidemia) was defined (Fig. 5). Within this syndrome, it was also soon apparent that not all patients had hyperglycinemia (Nyhan et al., 1972). Further research into propionic acidemia has also resulted in a subdivision of the syndrome. Primarily based on data from complementation studies, it has been possible to define three types of propionyl CoA carboxylase defects viz: pCCA, pCCB and pCCC (Gravel *et al.*, 1977). The occurrence of hyperglycinemia within this group of inherited defects does not correlate with any of the complementation groups.

3.3.2.3 Other organic acidemias sometimes presenting with hyperglycinemia

Hyperglycinemia has been seen in cases of other inborn defects, namely β-ketothiolase deficiency (Keating *et al.*, 1972) and isovaleryl-CoA dehydrogenase deficiency (Ando *et al.*, 1971 A; Saudubray *et al.*, 1976). As seen in Fig. 5, the defects are localized in the degradation pathways of isoleucine and valine respectively. In both syndromes, hyperglycinemia is rare. It was found in only one out of thirteen cases of β-ketothiolase deficiency and in two out of about fifty cases of isovaleryl-CoA dehydrogenase deficiency. In the case described by Ando *et al.* (1971 A), the abnormality in glycine oxidation was far less pronounced than that seen in cases of propionic acidemia with hyperglycinemia.

3.3.2.4 The etiology of the hyperglycinemia found in patients with inherited organic acidemias

The first real breakthrough in attempts to demonstrate the defect that directly causes the hyperglycinemia seen in patients with "ketotic" hyperglycinemia, came from the Japanese group which had characterized the glycine cleavage system. As early as 1969, Tada and coworkers (Tada *et al.*, 1969) measured the glycine cleavage activity in a liver biopsy from a patient with hyperglycinemia, who later turned out to have propionic acidemia (Nischimura *et al.*, 1974). They demonstrated a diminished $^{14}CO_2$-production in incubations with both ^{14}C-1-glycine and ^{14}C-2-glycine. Investigations of the degree of labelling of serine in these incubations revealed that the incorporation of ^{14}C into serine from ^{14}C-2-glycine was equal to the incorporation of ^{14}C into serine from ^{14}C-1-glycine. Normally this ratio is close to 2:1 (see Fig. 2). In this patient, the glycine cleavage activity was therefore clearly diminished.

In patients with methylmalonic acidemia and hyperglycinemia, similar results were obtained (Tada *et al.*, 1974). Furthermore, serine hydroxymethyl transferase activity in liver tissue was normal (Tada *et al.* 1974). The underlying cause for hyperglycinemia in both propionic acidemia and methylmalonic acidemia is therefore probably a diminished glycine cleavage activity. The same Japanese group later demonstrated that this change is mainly caused by lower H-protein activity, perhaps due to reduced synthesis (Hayasaka *et al.*, 1982).

These investigations clearly indicated that the glycine cleavage system was defective in "ketotic" hyperglycinemia. From the available knowledge an interrelationship between the degradation of the branched-chain amino acid and the glycine cleavage system was, however, not expected. The first indication for such an interaction was given by Hayasaka and co-workers (Hayasaka *et al.*, 1982). They investigated a patient with propionic acidemia, who had previously had hyperglycinemia. Because of treatment with a low-protein diet, this patient was clinically stable at the time of investigation. Glycine concentrations were then normal as was the glycine cleavage activity in liver tissue. From these findings, it was concluded that the glycine cleavage deficiency was reversible and therefore probably secondary, and that it varied with the severity of the derangement in propionic acid metabolism.

A number of model experiments have been performed in an attempt to elucidate a possible relationship between the branched-chain amino acid metabolism and the glycine cleavage system. Hillman and co-workers (Hillman *et al.*, 1973; Hillman and Otto, 1974) investigated glycine metabolism in fibroblasts from their patients with β-ketothiolase deficiency and hyperglycinemia. Glycine metabolism was studied by measuring the $^{14}CO_2$ production after incubation of intact fibroblasts with ^{14}C-U-glycine. The incorporation of ^{14}C into serine was also measured in experiments with fibroblast homogenates in a reaction medium containing NAD, pyridoxal phosphate, THF (cofactors for the glycine cleavage system and not for serine hydroxymethyl transferase) and either ^{14}C-1-glycine or ^{14}C-2-glycine. In these experiments, they demonstrated substantial $^{14}CO_2$ production and ^{14}C labelling in serine in normal fibroblasts. These workers suggest that the following phenomena were demonstrated: 1, A slightly diminished $^{14}CO_2$ production and serine labelling in the patient's cells compared to that in control cells; 2, Inhibition of the glycine degradation in cells from the patient after incubation and preincubation with isoleucine. This inhibition was not seen in control cells; 3, Normalisation of the glycine to serine transformation after dialysis of cell homogenate, suggesting the existence of a low molecular weight inhibitor. In a separate series Hillman and co-workers suggested tiglic acid to be this low molecular weight inhibitor. However, there are great difficulties in evaluating these results, since other workers could not demonstrate a glycine cleavage activity in fibroblasts at all (Kølvraa, 1979).

O'Brien (1978) has also studied the influence of metabolites from the branched-chain amino acids on the glycine cleavage system. He investigated a number of metabolites for inhibitory effect on the intact mitochondrial glycine cleavage system and found that the three primary transamination products (2-oxo-isovaleric acid, 2-oxo-3-methyl-valeric acid and 2-oxo-isocaproic acid) inhibited glycine cleavage moderately. Neither tiglic acid nor free CoA were inhibitory. Further studies revealed that the oxo-acids were oxidized during the incubation and that an increase in oxo-acid concentration in the incubations resulted in the inhibition increasing up to only about 50%.

O'Brien considered these findings to be the results of inhibition of the glycine cleavage system by the branched-chain oxo-acids themselves. However, the lack of inhibition beyond 50% with increasing inhibitor concentration seems strongly to indicate that the oxo-acids must first be metabolized into active

27

inhibitors. Furthermore, it is important to note that hyperglycinemia is not seen in maple syrup urine disease, which is characterized by an accumulation of branched-chain oxoacids. The findings of O'Brien thus support the hypothesis that one or more of the metabolites of the branched-chain amino acid degradation inhibit the glycine cleavage system, but the identity of the inhibitor has not been determined.

Kølvraa (1979) performed a more systematic investigation on the effect of almost all metabolites from the degradation of branched-chain amino acids and of several detoxification products from accumulated metabolites on rat liver glycine cleavage system. Significant inhibition of the system by 2-oxo-isovaleric acid, 2-methylbutyric acid and isobutyric acid was demonstrated. The first two to three metabolites in the degradation pathway of each of the three branched-chain amino acids had no effect on the glycine cleavage activity, while metabolites such as propionic acid, methylmalonic acid, 3-hydroxy-isobutyric acid, 2-methyl-3-hydroxy-butyric acid and tiglic acid exhibited a slight (10% - 25%) stimulating effect (Kølvraa unpublished). This stimulation was not investigated further but it seems consistent with the "propionic acid effect" described by Hampton and co-workers (Hampton *et al.*, 1983; 1984). Kølvraa (1979) continued to investigate the effect of 2-oxo-isovaleric acid, 2-methylbutyric acid and isobutyric acid on solubilized rat liver glycine cleavage system. The author demonstrated that the observed inhibition was probably caused by inhibition of the glycine cleavage system by 2-methylbutyryl-CoA (K_i 0.2-0.3 mmol/l) and isobutyryl-CoA (K_i 0.1-0.15 mmol/l). These two compounds therefore fulfill the criteria for being *in vivo* glycine cleavage inhibitors.

Haysaka and Tada (1983) extended their investigations to isovaleryl-CoA, tiglyl-CoA, propionyl-CoA, methylmalonyl-CoA and succinyl-CoA. They demonstrated substantial inhibition by all CoA-derivatives on the glycine cleavage activity, but only isovaleryl-CoA, tiglyl-CoA and isobutyryl-CoA inhibited the $^{14}CO_2$ exchange reaction. Furthermore it was demonstrated, at least with tiglyl-CoA as inhibitor, that the inhibition was caused mainly by competitive inhibition of the P-protein by H-protein.

In conclusion, all inhibition studies suggest that inhibition of the glycine cleavage system *in vivo* can be caused by saturated as well as unsaturated short- and branched-chain acyl-CoA's.

Of special interest in this connection is the anti-epileptic drug dipropyl-acetate (DPA). Children treated with this drug often exhibit hyperglycinuria and alaninuria (Jaeken *et al.*, 1977). This finding has been studied in detail by several groups in an attempt to elucidate the etiology behind "ketotic" hyperglycinemia. DPA-administration to rats causes both hyperglycinemia and hyperglycinuria (Mortensen *et al.*, 1980; Cherruau *et al.*, 1981) and the hyperglycinuria is dosedependent (Mortensen, 1980). DPA-treated rats have a diminished glycine cleavage activity (Kochi *et al.*, 1979; Mortensen *et al.*, 1980) and the glycine cleavage system in liver mitochondria is inhibited by DPA

(Kochi *et al.*, 1979; Mortensen *et al.*, 1980), and especially by DPA-CoA (Mortensen *et al.*, 1980). Kochi *et al.*, (1979), have also investigated which compound of the glycine cleavage system is diminished. By purifying the liver enzyme complex both from DPA treated rats and normal rats they demonstrated a decrease of the P-protein but not of the H-protein. Furthermore, the results suggested an inhibition of enzyme synthesis together with inhibited enzyme activity in DPA-treated rats.

The DPA effect therefore shows substantial analogies with inhibitions of the glycine cleavage system caused by short- and branched-chain acyl-CoA's. However, the various acyl-CoA's probably inhibit the P-protein and it is the H-protein that is diminished in propionic and methylmalonic acidurias.

3.3.2.5   Conclusion

It can be concluded that when hyperglycinemia occurs in connection with inborn errors in the degradation of branched-chain amino acids, it is caused by diminished glycine cleavage activity. The normalisation of the glycine cleavage activity by therapeutic control of the primary enzyme defect is compatible with the hypothesis that an inhibitor derived from the primary defect inhibits synthesis and/or activity of one or more compounds in the glycine cleavage system.

A number of observations suggest that short- and branched-chain acyl-CoA's are responsible for the inhibition. It remains to be proven whether one or more of these possible candidates actually accumulate sufficiently intracellularly to cause *in vivo* inhibition.

3.3.3   Nonketotic hyperglycinemia

A description of the first case of nonketotic hyperglycinemia was published in 1965 by Gerritsen and co-workers. Since then, more than 100 patients with this disease have been described. The disease shows far less variation in its biochemical and clinical aspects than "ketotic" hyperglycinemias. A large number of cases have been found in Finland. Von Wendt has evaluated all cases up to 1980 (Von Wendt 1980).

Diagnostic biochemical criteria are:

1. Hyperglycinuria: 5-20 times normal
2. Hyperglycinemia: 3-10 times normal
3. High glycine concentration in cerebrospinal fluid. (Other groups have stressed that the ratio of cerebrospinal fluid-glycine:serum-glycine is diagnostic. In nonketotic hyperglycinemia it is between 0.2 - 0.3, while in normal individuals it is between 0.02 - 0.03 (Perry *et al.*, 1975)).
4. Abnormal response to glycine loading.
5. Diminished glycine cleavage activity.
6. Normal excretion of organic acids in urine.
7. No metabolic acidosis or ketosis.

The diagnosis cannot be made on clinical symptoms alone since all symptoms are fairly nonspecific. The Finnish group (Von Wendt and Similä, 1982) has tried to define three subgroups, mainly based on the time of presentation.

A. Neonatal type

This type seems to be the most common, comprising about 2/3 of all cases. Clinical symptoms such as hypotonia, lethargy and difficulties with feeding, begin within a few hours after birth (Brun *et al.*, 1979) or as late as one week after birth (Similä and Visakorpi, 1970; Bernardina *et al.*, 1979; Kølvraa *et al.*, 1979). Based on biochemical, pathological and EEG-investigations it seems, however, that the condition has already manifested itself before birth (de Groot *et al.*, 1977; Brun *et al.*, 1979; Von Wendt *et al.*, 1981). Apart from the initial hypotonia, the clinical picture is dominated by rapid deterioration with myoclonia and frequently depression of respiration necessitating assisted ventilation (Carson, 1982). If the patients survive the neonatal period, spontaneous respiration returns despite of continuous high glycine values, and the children can be extubated (Kølvraa *et al.*, 1979; de Groot *et al.*, 1978). Altogether, about 50% of the patients survive the neonatal period (Carsen, 1982), but they are severely mentally retarded and often die later in childhood due to general complications.

B. The infantile type

Von Wendt (1980) has defined a group of patients in which the onset of symptoms starts later in the first year of life. Apart from this, the symptomes are the same as in the neonatal type. It is arguable whether the differentiation of this type from the neonatal type serves any useful purpose.

C. Late onset type

This type is clearly distinct, due to its late age of onset (from 2 years of age, to even as late as post-school-age). These patients generally survive with

30

rather moderate intellectual dysfunctions and present a very heterogeneous picture, especially regarding the neurological symptoms. At present, only 15 patients of this type have been described. The clinical picture varies substantially within this group, from severe mental retardation (Flannery *et al.*, 1983) to normal mental developement (Banks and Morrow, 1972).

While the clinical picture thus varies considerably, the biochemical parameters show far less variation. However, it should be stressed that most of these investigations have been performed on patients with the neonatal type. The dominant biochemical finding is one of isolated elevation in glycine concentration in body fluids. Especially the concentration of glycine in cerebrospinal fluid has been investigated in detail because of the neuro-transmitter function of glycine. The cerebrospinal fluid concentration of glycine is normally kept extremely low ($< 10 \ \mu mol/l$) by the two transport systems (Davidoff and Adair, 1975; Balcar and Johnstons, 1973). As a result, a very pronounced concentration gradient exists between cerebrospinal fluid and both blood (normal blood glycine concentration $= 300 \ \mu mol/l$) and the intracellular fluid in the central nervous system (normal glycine concentration intracellularly $= 2000$-$7000 \ \mu mol/l$) (Perry *et al.*, 1977). The characteristic finding in nonketotic hyperglycinemia is that these two gradients have partly disappeared due to a very pronounced increase in the glycine concentration in the cerebrospinal fluids compared to that in blood. On this background, several groups have investigated glycine transport across cell membranes in patients with nonketotic hyperglycinemia. Initially, data were presented indicating that the cell membrane transport of glycine was diminished in cultured fibroblasts from patients with nonketotic hyperglycinemia (Revsin and Morrow, 1976). Later, however, several groups (Halton and Krieger, 1980; Kelly *et al.*, 1979; Kølvraa *et al.*, 1983) demonstrated that glycine transport is normal. The break-down in the concentration gradient found in patients with nonketotic hyperglycinemia is probably caused solely by the very pronounced glycine accumulation, especially in the central nervous system (4-10 times normal (Perry *et al.*, 1977)). Since the high affinity uptake process has a rather low capacity, accumulations of this magnitude would be expected to saturate the system. This would result in an increase in the glycine concentration in cerebrospinal fluid, up to a level where the low affinity process works optimally.

The site of the causal defect in patients with nonketotic hyperglycinemia has been located in the glycine cleavage system. This was clearly indicated by the original studies on *in vivo* oxidation of ^{14}C-1-glycine and ^{14}C-2-glycine performed by Ando and co-workers (Ando *et al.*, 1968). Others have demonstrated a diminished glycine cleavage activity, firstly in liver tissue (de Groot *et al.*, 1970; Kølvraa *et al.*, 1979) and later, in cerebral tissue (Perry *et al.*, 1977). While a certain activity (from 10 - 50% of normal) can be demonstrated in liver tissue from the patients, the lack of glycine cleavage activity in the central nervous system seems to be almost total.

The Japanese group of Kikuchi has tried to determine which of the compounds

31

of the glycine cleavage system is defective in liver tissue from patients with nonketotic hyperglycinemia. In three patients, whose post mortem liver and brain tissue were investigated for P, H and T-protein, this group surprisingly demonstrated three different defects. In a patient with a slightly atypical picture (progressive neurodegeneration after a period of normal development) a severe deficiency of H-protein activity was demonstrated both in liver and brain tissue. This was probably caused by the fact that H-protein did not contain lipoic acid (Hiraga et al., 1981). At the same time, a slightly diminished P-protein activity was found. In another patient an isolated decrease in P-protein activity was demonstrated, probably caused by lack of the enzyme protein (Hayasaka et al., 1983). In the last patient a severe diminution in T-protein activity has been demonstrated (Hayasaka et. al. 1983). The syndrome of nonketotic hyperglycinemia thus seems genetically heterogeneous, since the same glycine cleavage deficiency can be caused by genetic defects in at least three of the four compounds in the glycine cleavage system.

Very little is known about the consequences of glycine cleavage deficiency and the resulting glycine accumulation. One feature, however, is striking. The symptoms in patients with nonketotic hyperglycinemia are predominantly cerebral, while the symptoms in patients with "ketotic" hyperglycinemia are more generalized, without pronounced involvement of the central nervous system. This is compatible with the observations found by Perry and co-workers (Perry et al., 1977). They showed that patients with nonketotic hyperglycinemia have severely diminished glycine cleavage activity in brain tissue but only moderately diminished liver glycine cleavage activity, while patients with "ketotic" hyperglycinemia have diminished activity of the glycine cleavage system in liver tissue, but normal activity in brain tissue and normal glycine concentrations in cerebrospinal fluid. These facts clearly suggest that the central nervous system is the organ primary affected in nonketotic hyperglycinemia.

\The pathological features in patients with nonketotic hyperglycinemia should thus primarily be found in the central nervous system. Several groups of workers have investigated the changes in the central nervous system. A certain demyelination, combined with spongiosis of the white substance in several areas of the central nervous system (especially cerebellum, the brain stem and medulla spinalis) have generally been found, while no abnormalities in the peripheral nerves occured (Brun et al., 1979; Agamanolis et al., 1982). The vacuoles found in the white substance are comprised of myeline lamellae without cellular covering - abnormalities that are also seen in a number of other amino acidemias (Agamanolis et al., 1982). Furthermore, varying degrees of astrocytgliosis have been described (Agamanolis et. al. 1982).

The primary hypotonia, which develops within the first week of life, has previously been attributed to excessive postsynaptic inhibition by increased glycine concentration in cerebrospinal fluid (Kølvraa et al., 1979). However, the modest effect of strychnine treatment in these patients (von Wendt, 1980), suggests that other mechanisms occure quite early, perhaps including structural damage to the myelin. Such structural damage can probably explain all the less specific neurological symptomes that occure later, symptoms which also occur in patients with other amino acidemias, e.g. phenylketonuria, maple syrup urine disease and homocystinuria.

The occurrence of structural damage in the central nervous system early in the course of the disease, may also explain the lack of effect of treatment. A number of different therapeutic principles have been tried. These include attempts to deplete the body of glycine using such methods as diet, increased glycine conjugation, exchange transfusions and peritonial dialysis (Baumgarth et al., 1969; Leupold et al., 1974; Kølvraa et al., 1979; Carson, 1982). The effect of administration of C_1-fragments (methionine, leucovorine, formate, choline) has also been studied (Trijbels et al., 1974; Kølvraa et al., 1979; Carson, 1982), as well as attempts to modify the neurophysiological effect of glycine using strychnine and benzodiazepam, or by the installation of a shunt between the cerebrospinal fluid and blood (Kriger et al., 1977; Gitzelman et al., 1977; MacDermot et al., 1980; Matalon et al., 1983).

These attempts at treatment sometimes resulted in partial normalization of the biochemical parameters, but no alteration in the clinical course of the disease occurred.

33

4. THE SYNDROME D-GLYCERIC ACIDEMIA WITH HYPERGLYCINEMIA

4.1 CLINICAL PICTURE

The patient (A.J.), a boy, was born in 1972. The parents were unrelated immigrants from Serbia (Brandt et al., 1974; Brandt et al., 1976; Kølvraa et al., 1976). The patient had one elder brother who was normal. Pregnancy and delivery were uncomplicated, weight at birth was 3350 g, length 52 cm. Immediately after birth it was noticed that the patient was extremely hypotonic and had difficulties with feeding. After 8 weeks, general seizures occurred. After that the boy did not develop mentally at all. During the following years several types of seizures developed, such as myoclonic jerks, cerebellar attacks and periodically, an almost classical chorea minor. Persistent anti-epileptic treatment was given, which could only partially control the seizures. The patient died in status epilepticus at the age of 3 1/2 years.

A detailed family history could not be obtained, since the mother was killed in a traffic accident when the child was about one year old, and the father then left the country together with the elder brother.

4.2 GENERAL LABORATORY INVESTIGATIONS

During the various admissions, routine laboratory tests were always normal. In particular, no tendency to ketosis or acidosis was demonstrated. Initial measurements of mannosidase, galactosidase, galactosaminidase and alkaline phosphatase were performed on leucocytes and found to be normal. Arylsulphatase A excretion in urine was normal, as was the excretion of hexosamine and glucuronic acid. The karyotype was normal. The only abnormal laboratory findings were slightly elevated concentrations of aspartate aminotransferase, 2-hydroxybutyrate dehydrogenase and alkaline phosphatase in serum.

4.3 METABOLIC SCREENING

The patient's body fluids were screened for metabolic abnormalities when he was one week old. At this time, investigation of amino acids in urine using thin-layer chromatography was performed and a very strong spot at the location of glycine was demonstrated. Quantitative amino acid analysis was then performed on both blood and urine and later on spinal fluid. In this way a pronounced accumulation of glycine was demonstrated in blood (0.3-1.5 mmol/l), spinal fluid (0.12 mmol/l) and urine (22-61 mmol/l)(Table 1).

Table 1.

HABITUAL VARIATION IN URINARY EXCRETION (μmol/24 h) OF A NUMBER OF RELEVANT COMPOUNDS.

The pattern of excretion in patient A.J. was compared to the pattern of excretion in patients with indicated defects in the glycine metabolism (I), in the metabolism of D-glyceric acid (II) and in the metabolism of acyl-CoA's (III).

Compound	A.J.	I. Nonketotic hyperglycinemia (Kolvraa et al. 1979).	II. D-glyceric acidemia		III. Riboflavin responsive acyl-CoA dehydrogenation deficiency (Gregersen et al. 1982)	Controls
			Wadman et al. 1976.	Duran et al. 1988		
A. Glycine	$25\text{-}85 \times 10^3$	$3\text{-}25 \times 10^3$	<5	<5	<5	<5
B. D-glyceric acid	$8\text{-}20 \times 10^3$	<500	$4\text{-}8 \times 10^3$	$1\text{-}10 \times 10^3$	<500	<500
C. Isobutyrylglycine	1-10	<2[a]	-	-	10-30	< 0.1
2-Me-butyrylglycine	0.5-10	<1[a]	-	-	0-4	< 0.1
isovalerylglycine	0.5-30	<1[a]	-	-	10-35	< 0.4
butyrylglycine	0-10	<1[a]	-	-	0-3	< 0.1
hexanoylglycine	1-3	<1[a]	-	-	75-125	< 0.1
adipic acid	< 2	-	-	-	300-600	< 10
suberic acid	6-15	-	-	-	50-100	< 3
sebasic acid	< 1	-	-	-	20-75	< 3

[a] measured on a AEI MS 30 mass spectrometer, which had a rather low resolution and therefore higher limit of detection.

Screening for organic acids in urine using gas chromatography, demonstrated the presence of an abnormal compound in substantial amounts (Kølvraa et al., 1976). Using mass spectometry, this compound was identified as glyceric acid. Since glyceric acid can occur as both the D- and L-isomer, its configuration was investigated. This was done after isolation of the compound using ionexchange chromatography. Firstly, enzymatic investigations were performed based on the principle that lactate dehydrogenase has affinity only towards the L-form while D-glycerate dehydrogenase only has affinity towards the D-form. Later, the optical rotation dispersion was investigated. Using both these methods, it was demonstrated that the glyceric acid excreted by the patient was of the D-isomer form. Further investigations demonstrated the presence of glyceric acid in serum (the concentration ranging from 1.0 - 1.3 mmol/l) Quantities of D-glyceric acid in urine ranged from 14 - 23 mmol/24 hours (Table 1).

The gas chromatographic/mass spectrometric analysis of urine also demonstrated a constant excretion of a number of metabolites which are known to be derived from branched- and straight-chain acyl-CoA's (Table 1). The excretion of propionic acid and methylmalonic acid was normal.

4.4 STUDIES ON THE METABOLIC DERANGEMENTS

Metabolic studies on this patient demonstrated severe accumulation of two different metabolites, namely glycine and D-glyceric acid. Both accumulations were very pronounced. Glycine accumulation was comparable to that found in patients with nonketotic hyperglycinemia, while D-glyceric acid accumulation was comparable to that found in the two patients with D-glyceric acidemia described by the Dutch group (Wadman et al., l976; Duran et al., 1988).

Our investigations on the causal metabolic defect (or defects) included attempts to demonstrate a connection between the glycine and the D-glyceric acid accumulation as well as separate studies on each accumulation. Regarding the metabolites derived from acyl-CoA's, it was evident that the amounts excreted were small compared to glycine and D-glyceric acid, and a primary enzyme defect was therefore unlikely. Nevertheless, the metabolism of straight- and branched-chain acyl-CoA's was investigated, since these acyl-CoA's have been implicated in the "secondary" hyperglycinemia seen in propionic acidemia and methylmalonic acidemia. These studies are presented in section 4.4.2.

4.4.1 The metabolism of glycine and of D-glyceric acid

4.4.1.1 Interconversion between glycine and D-glyceric acid

The biochemical relationship between glycine and D-glyceric acid can be seen in Fig. 1. It does not seem probable that glycine was formed in significant amounts from D-glyceric acid, since intravenous administration of ^{14}C-1-glyceric acid to

36

the patient did not give detectable labelling of glycine (Kølvraa et al., 1980 B). Formation of D-glyceric acid from glycine cannot be excluded with the same certainty, however, since the reverse tracer experiment, where ^{14}C-1-glycine was administered, resulted in a weak labelling (below 2% of the dose administered) of glyceric acid and of serine. The labelling was, however, so slight that it was probably a result of modest glycine oxidation with concomitant low, diffuse labelling of both glucose and fructose and the final trapping of some radioactive carbon-atoms in D-glyceric acid.

In this context, it is relevant that a significant decrease in excretion of both glycine and serine caused by a glycine-serine-proline-free diet did not alter the amounts of D-glyceric acid excreted (Kølvraa et al., 1984).

Another argument against the hypothesis that D-glyceric acid might be formed from primarily accumulated glycine is that D-glyceric acid accumulation is not seen in the condition nonketotic hyperglycinemia (Kølvraa et al., 1979).

4.4.1.2   Glycine metabolism in the patient

In an attempt to elucidate the etiology of the glycine accumulation, a number of investigations have been performed; investigations which correspond to those done in patients with nonketotic hyperglycinemia, namely: *in vivo* and *in vitro* oxidation of radioactive glycine (Kølvraa et al., 1980 B). The membrane transport of glycine in cultured fibroblasts was also investigated (Kølvraa et al., 1983).

In vivo glycine oxidation was investigated by monitoring the excretion of ^{14}CO$_2$ after intravenous injection of labelled glycine. It was demonstrated that the patient had a very low oxidation rate of radioactive glycine, similar to the rate seen in patients with nonketotic hyperglycinemia. However as earlier described, an experiment of this type is hampered by the fact that patients have an increased glycine pool which can result in too low an estimate of the degradation rate, compared to controls.

Furthermore, the glycine cleavage system was measured in postmortem liver tissue from the patient and compared to tissue activity in three controls. A substantial decrease was demonstrated, down to 10% of normal (Kølvraa et al., 1980 B). The glycine transport across cell membranes in cultured fibroblasts was also measured and found normal (Kølvraa et al., 1983). In conclusion, it seems evident that the glycine accumulation is due to a defective glycine cleavage reaction.

It may be expected that the other available degradation pathways would prevent accumulation of glycine, so it is surprising that this patient and others with hyperglycinemia due to diminished glycine cleavage activity, had such severe glycine accumulation. As described earlier, it seems, however, that only conversion to serine and possibly glycine conjugation could play a role in avoiding glycine accumulation. The amounts of glycine which are excreted as acylglycines in various types of hyperglycinemia are negligible, however (Kølvraa et al., 1980 A; Bartlett and Gompertz, 1974; Sweetman et al., 1978). With regards to serine hydroxymethyl transferase-catalysis it is evident that the degradation of glycine via this pathway does not operate in these patients. This is shown, firstly because patients with hyperglycinemia can have 6-7 times normal glycine concentrations in blood without concomitant serine accumulation and secondly, because injections of large doses of glycine did not cause a rise in the concentration of serine in a patient with late onset nonketotic hyperglycinemia (Steiman et al., 1979). The answer probably lies in the role of the CH_2-THF in the serine-glycine interconversion. As previously mentioned, the glycine cleavage reaction is considered to be the most important reaction for production of CH_2-THF. Since the glycine cleavage system and serine hydroxymethyl transferase are located in the same mitochondrial compartment (Motokawa and Kikuchi, 1971), it seems possible that the CH_2-THF's produced by glycine cleavage are primarily used in the serine hydroxymethyl transferase-catalysed reaction (Arnstein and Neuberg, 1953). This would create a situation where diminished glycine cleavage activity "locks" both reactions. It thus seems probable that, despite its complex biochemistry, glycine accumulation can be fully explained only by diminished glycine cleavage. Finally, it should be noted that neither D-glyceric acid nor D-glyceraldehyde inhibited the glycine cleavage system in rat liver mitochondria (Kølvraa et al., 1980 B and unpublished).

4.4.1.3   The metabolism of D-glyceric acid in the patient

Based on detailed studies of the excretion pattern, it was originally thought that the enzyme defect was localized at the level of the D-glycerate dehydrogenase (Kølvraa et al., 1976). The activity of this enzyme was subsequently measured and found to be reduced to 25 % of normal (Kølvraa et al., 1976). Mixing experiments with homogenate from patient and control showed a full additive effect. In spite of several attempts, it turned out to be impossible to demonstrate D-glycerate kinase activity either in leucocytes or fibroblasts from normal persons, and this enzyme was therefore never measured in the patient.

Based on these findings, we initially assumed that the patient had an inherited deficiency of D-glycerate dehydrogenase. However, there were grounds for reconsidering this assumption. At the time of the investigation the results from Williams and Smith (1968 A) were available, demonstrating that the patients with L-glyceric acidemia had an identical enzyme deficiency (diminished D-glycerate dehydrogenase activity), but exhibited a different clinical and biochemical picture. Later information concerning two other patients with D-glyceric acidemia showed that at least the patient described by Wadman et al. (1976) must be considered to have normal D-glycerate dehydrogenase activity and yet, in spite of this, the patient excreted substantial amounts of D-glyceric acid.

38

Due to these inconsistencies, we performed *in vivo* loading tests in an attempt to get a broader picture of the metabolic derangement of D-glyceric acid (Kølvraa *et al.*, 1984). Two compounds are relevant in such loading tests, namely serine and fructose (se section 2.1). Due to the fact that patients with nonketotic hyperglycinemia show intolerance towards serine, we did not perform a loading test with this compound. In a therapeutic trial where the patient was treated with a glycine-serine-proline-free diet, a significant reduction in serine excretion did not result in any alteration in D-glyceric acid excretion. This finding seems to suggest that serine is not a major precursor of D-glyceric acid in the patient. Loading tests with fructose was performed when the patient was 18 months old (Kølvraa *et al.*, 1984). Two loading tests were performed with a four week interval between the two, first with 6 g fructose and later with 12 g fructose. In the following 24 hours, urine was collected and D-glyceric acid was measured. In the month prior to the loading tests, five urine samples were collected in order to determine the habitual excretion level. These investigations showed that fructose administration caused a substantial increase in the excretion of D-glyceric acid. On administration of 12 g fructose, a statistically significant increase resulted. If all the fructose administered was to be metabolized exclusively through the pathway involving D-glyceric acid, about 50% of the dose could be converted to D-glyceric acid. Within the first 24 hours after administration of 12 g fructose, the increase in excretion of D-glyceric acid was as much as 3.8 g, indicating that fructose must be a major precursor of D-glyceric acid.

With regards to the normal metabolism of D-glyceraldehyde in the "D-glyceraldehyde crossroad", these findings seem to indicate a metabolic defect localized in the degradation of fructose, possibly at the level of D-glyceraldehyde. This might cause an abnormal shunting of D-glyceraldehyde into D-glyceric acid. The accumulation of D-glyceric acid is then probably due to the fact that transformation of D-glyceraldehyde to D-glyceric acid in man is a blind alley (Heinz *et al.*, 1968). Further support for this hypothesis would require liver or kidney tissues from the patient. Unfortunately no kidney tissue and only enough liver tissue for glycine cleavage determination was obtained postmortally and therefore detailled studies of the fructose degradation have not been performed.

It can therefore be concluded that the cause of the D-glyceric acid accumulation is still unclear, but that available data seem to indicate a derangement in fructose degradation. The moderately diminished D-glycerate dehydrogenase activity in leucocytes from the patient could be explained by the fact that this enzyme is under strict metabolic control and is regulated both by fructose and glucose metabolites.

4.4.1.4   Conclusion
The data obtained to date suggest the existence of two different enzyme deficiencies with concomitant accumulations. No data connecting these two deficiencies have been obtained so far, apart from the fact that fluctuations in

the two accumulations occure in concert with one another most of the time (Kølvraa *et al.*, 1980 B). This correlation may, however, be due to more general fluctuations in the patients overall metabolism, fluctuations which can occur as a result of slight starvation, intercurrent disease etc.

4.4.2 The metabolism of acyl-CoA's in the patient

4.4.2.1 The normal metabolism of acyl-CoA's

A short review of the normal metabolism of straight- and branched-chain acyl-CoA's will be given before the experiments performed in order to elucidate the metabolism of these compounds in A.J. are presented.

Medium-chain acyl-CoA's occur as intermediates in the normal β-oxidation of long-chain fatty acids. These are shortened in length by successive removal of acetyl-CoA ending as acetyl-CoA. Furthermore, they occur in the degradation of the branched-chain amino acids leucine, isoleucine and valine which, after transamination and decarboxylation, are transformed to isovaleryl-CoA, 2-methylbutyryl-CoA and isobutyryl-CoA respectively (Fig. 5). The two following degradation steps are analogous for the straight-chain and branched-chain acyl-CoA's (apart from isovaleryl-CoA). These are dehydrogenation, catalyzed by acyl-CoA dehydrogenases, followed by hydroxylation catalyzed by an enoyl-CoA hydratase (Fig. 6).

Five distinct enzymes exist for the dehydrogenation of the various monocarboxyl-CoA's. Three have overlapping chain length affinities in the degradation of fatty acids (Ikeda *et al.*, 1985), one is a distinct isovaleryl-CoA dehydrogenase (Ikeda and Tanaka, 1983) and one is a common dehydrogenase for 2-methylbutyryl-CoA and isobutyryl-CoA (Ikeda and Tanaka, 1982). Common to all these dehydrogenases is the fact that they are flavoenzymes with FAD as the prostetic group. For all acyl-CoA dehydrogenases the hydrogen atoms formed are transfered from the FAD-group to the electron transfer flavoprotein (ETF), which transports the electrons via ETF dehydrogenase to the respiration chain (Fig. 6)(Hall, 1981; Ruzicka and Beinert, 1977; Rhead *et al.*, 1981).

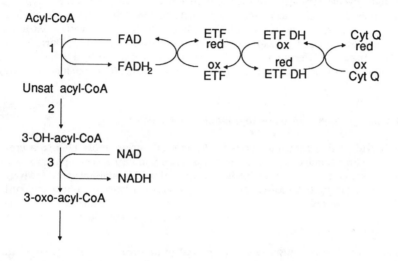

Fig. 6.   The β-oxidation cycle involved in the degradation of straight-chain acyl-CoA's, isobutyryl-CoA and 2-methyl-butyryl-CoA. 1.: acyl-CoA dehydrogenase; 2.: enoyl-CoA hydratase; 3.: 3-hydroxy-acyl-CoA dehydrogenase

4.4.2.2   Inherited defects in the acyl-CoA dehydrogenation

Until now, well-defined defects with characteristic metabolic profiles have been described in isovaleryl-CoA dehydrogenase (Rhead and Tanaka, 1980), medium-chain acyl-CoA dehydrogenase (Kølvraa et al., 1982) and long-chain acyl-CoA dehydrogenase (Hale et al., 1985). Furthermore, metabolic defects have been described which seem to be localized to either ETF or ETF dehydrogenase (Christensen et al., 1984; Frerman and Goodman, 1985).

The low molecular weight metabolites excreted in these various disorders include glycine conjugates of the accumulated acyl-CoA's for defects involving the branched-chain acyl-coA's. For defects involving the straight-chain acyl-CoA's, excreted metabolites include glycine conjugates, carnitine conjugates and C_6 - C_{10} dicarboxylic acids (Gregersen et al., 1983; Duran et al., 1985). In table 1, the amounts of these compounds excreted by a patient with a riboflavin responsive acyl-CoA dehydrogenation defect (Gregersen et. al. 1982) is shown.

4.4.2.3   Acyl-CoA dehydrogenation in the patient

It is evident that the compounds found in A.J's urine (table 1 C) to a great extent corresponded to the compounds found in urine from patients with inherited defects in the acyl-CoA dehydrogenation. The amounts excreted were, however, substantially lower. Never the less, A.J's urinary organic acid profile clearly suggested, that the rate of oxidation of branched-chain and straight-chain fatty acids was lower than normal, and that the ratelimiting step was at the level of the acyl-CoA dehydrogenases.

The diminished oxidation rate was verified in in vitro experiments. Here, the ability of intact fibroblasts from the patient to oxidize both straight-chain and branched-chain fatty acids, was investigated and a moderately diminished oxidation rate for all acids was demonstrated (table 2). The decrease in oxidation rate was significant at the 95% level for longer-chain fatty acids and for isovaleric acid.

Also in vivo tests were used to characterize the diminished fatty acid oxidation. In these experiments the effect of riboflavin, which is precursor for FAD, was investigated. 30 mg riboflavin was given perorally, three times per day, for four weeks to the patient. A blood sample was taken and 24 hour urine samples were collected after three weeks and after four weeks of treatment. These were analysed for amino acids and organic acids. The concentrations found were compared statistically with the concentrations obtained from a series of samples taken during the three months prior to the treatment. It was in these experiments demonstrated that riboflavin treatment caused a pronounced decrease in excretion of acylglycines (Kølvraa et al., 1984). This riboflavin responsiveness clearly verified that the ratelimiting step was at the level of the acyl-CoA dehydrogenases, since these are the only enzymes in the degradation of branched-chain and straight-chain fatty acids that have FAD as prostetic group.

42

Table 2.

β-OXIDATION IN FIBROBLASTS FROM PATIENT A.J. COMPARED TO CONTROLS.

Expressed in nmols fatty acid oxidized/mg protein/hour.

Substrate	Hexanoic acid	Octanoic acid	Decanoic acid	Lauric acid	Myristic acid	Palmitic acid	Isovaleric acid
CONTROLS							
mean	1.26	0.60	1.81	1.62	1.23	4.78	0.26
range	1.03-1.75	0.38-0.83	1.20-2.44	0.97-2.07	1.02-1.68	3.61-6.81	0.16-0.32
s.d.	0.29	0.20	0.50	0.45	0.27	1.0	0.06
N	6	6	6	5	5	6	6
Patient A.J.	1.04	0.43	1.54	0.76	0.45	1.63	0.11
p	$0.2 < p < 0.3$	$0.2 < p < 0.3$	$0.3 < p < 0.5$	$0.05 < p < 0.1$	$0.01 < p < 0.02$	$0.01 < p < 0.025$	$0.02 < p < 0.05$

Fibroblasts in monolayer were incubated with ^{14}C-1-acids for 45 minutes at 37°C. Then citrate buffer pH:2 was added and $^{14}CO_2$ was collected. After protein solubilisation using sodium hydroxyd the reaction mixture was precipitated with perchloric acid and radio-labelled, perchloric acid-soluble metabolites were counted in supernatants. The activity was calculated from the sum of the two products (Kølvraa et al., 1982).

In a separate experiment the acyl-CoA dehydrogenase activity in freeze-thawn fibroblasts was measured with hexanoyl-CoA, octanoyl-CoA and decanoyl-CoA as substrates and using a mass spectrometric assay. The activities measured were found to be normal as was the activity of the two reference enzymes lactate dehydrogenase and glutamate dehydrogenase. Similarly the ability of intact fibroblasts to transforme riboflavin to FMN and FAD was investigated using ^{14}C-2-riboflavin (Christensen et. al. 1984). These investigations demonstrated normal riboflavin metabolism in the patient.

In summary it can be concluded that a general diminution of acyl-CoA dehydrogenation rate has been indicated both *in vivo* and in intact cells from the patient. Compared to the findings in patients with primary defects in acyl-CoA dehydrogenation, the reduction seems, however, modest and is therefore probably not due to a primary defect. A possible explanation could be intracellular accumulation of an inhibitor derived either from D-glyceric acid metabolism or glycine metabolism. The fact that a similar reduction could not be demonstrated in disintegrated systems might support such an explanation.

4.4.2.4 The relationship between acyl-CoA dehydrogenation and the metabolism of D-glyceric acid and glycine

In vivo loading tests were initially used to investigate the relationship between the diminished acyl-CoA dehydrogenation and the disturbed metabolism of D-glyceric acid and glycine. An attempt to identify a possible relationship between the metabolisms of D-glyceric acid and acyl-CoA's was made by monitoring acylglycine excretion during fructose loading, and monitoring D-glyceric acid excretion during riboflavin treatment. It was found that fructose loading caused a significant increase in the excretion of all acylglycines (Kølvraa *et al.*, 1984). In contrast, a decrease in acylglycine excretion caused by riboflavin treatment did not alter D-glyceric acid excretion. These results suggest that deranged acyl-CoA metabolism is a secondary phenomenon and is probably caused by deranged D-glyceric acid metabolism.

In vitro systems were used in an attempt to obtain experimental support for this hypothesis. These experiments were based on the hypothesis that a metabolite from the D-glyceric acid metabolism would be accumulated and cause inhibition of acyl-CoA dehydrogenation processes. However, it was impossible to demonstrate that D-glyceric acid or D-glyceraldehyde inhibited acyl-CoA dehydrogenation. Both compounds were added, in concentrations up to 10 mmol/l, to reaction mixtures in both assays for acyl-CoA dehydrogenases with various substrates and to β-oxidation assays on intact rat liver mitochondria (Osmundsen and Bremer, 1977) without any apparent inhibition (Kølvraa *et al.*, 1984). In addition, intact fibroblasts (from patient or control), cultured in media containing D-glyceric acid and D-glyceraldehyde, did not exhibit a significant reduction of β-oxidation rates (measured with ^{14}C-1-lauric acid as substrate). D-glyceraldehyde was found to be strongly cytotoxic in these experiments. The identification of the endogeneous inhibitor, suggested above,

44

has thus not been made, but D-glyceraldehyde cannot be excluded as a candidate.

While D-glyceric acid excretion remained constant during riboflavin treatment, a significant fall in glycine accumulation was observed (Kølvraa *et al.*, 1984). Whether this effect is due to the glycine cleavage system being affected by accumulated acyl-CoA's, or whether the fall in glycine excretion is due to a more general effect of riboflavin is unclear.

4.4.2.5   Conclusion
The diminution of acyl-CoA dehydrogenation, indicated in both *in vivo* and *in vitro* studies in patient A.J., is very modest compared to what is found in inherited defects in fatty acid oxidation. *In vivo* loading tests with fructose suggests that the diminution is secondary to the deranged fructose metabolism.

5. CONCLUDING REMARKS

The hyperglycinemia found in patient A.J. was investigated in detail. Clinically it is evident, that the picture corresponded closely to what is seen in the syndrome nonketotic hyperglycinemia. On the biochemical side all the criteria listed for the diagnosis nonketotic hyperglycinemia (p. 30) was investigated, except for the effect of a glycine load. Among these criterias only one was not fulfilled, namely that the excretion of organic acids should be normal. Here the patient A.J. deviated from the syndrome nonketotic hyperglycinemia in the fact, that he excreted elevated amounts of both D-glyceric acid (table 1 B) and a number of metabolites derived from accumulated acyl-CoA's (table 1C).

Also the accumulation of D-glyceric acid was investigated both *in vivo* and in *in vitro* systems and the results compared to what was found in other patients with D-glyceric acidemia. In our patient the excretion of D-glyceric acid was slightly higher, but in the same range, as in the two Dutch patients, of which the patient described by Duran *et al.* (1988) had a clinical picture very similar to A.J. The patient described by Wadman *et al.* (1976) had an entirely different picture. Also *in vivo* loading tests gave similar results in A.J. and Durans patient, namely increased excretion of D-glyceric acid after fructose loading. Serine seemed not to be a precursor of D-glyceric acid. Loading tests on Wadmans patient gave the reverse results. These results clearly suggested, that A.J. and Durans patient have the same or very similar defects, probably located in the degradation of fructose. A number of enzyme assays were performed on both A.J. and on Durans patient. In A.J. D-glycerate dehydrogenase was measured on leucocyte homogenate. These investigations revealed a reduction in activity down to 25% of normal controls. This result is, however, difficult to interpret. Firstly it may seem unlikely, considering the very severe accumulation of D-glyceric acid, that such a high residual activity would be found, if the D-glycerate dehydrogenase diminution was the primary defect. Secondly it is disturbing that patients with L-glyceric acidemia have undetectable activity of the same enzyme but an entirely different clinical picture.

Considering the various pathways from the "glyceraldehyd crossroad", a defect in triokinase may seem more probable. This enzyme was not measured in A.J., but it has been measured in erytrocytes from Durans patient and found normal. Whether this finding totally excludes a defect in f. ex. liver triokinase is, however, debatable. All in all it seems resonable to conclude that A.J. and Durans patient has the same or a very similar disturbance in the metabolism of fructose. The exact enzyme location remains, however, unknown.

At this point the simplest explanation of the excretion pattern in A.J. would be that he suffered from two independent i.e.o.m., namely nonketotic hyperglycinemia and an inherited defect in the metabolism of fructose similar to Durans patient.

46

The probability for the same child having two rare i.e.o.m. at the same time is, however, so low that the possibility of a causal link between them had to be considered. This possibility was investigated in a number of experiments. Firstly it was documented that conversion between glycine and D-glyceric acid was very low in A.J., thereby rejecting the hypothesis that one of the accumulated compounds was a metabolic product of the other. Secondly it was shown that D-glyceric acid did not inhibit the glycine cleavage system, an observation which is supported by the fact that none of the other patients with accumulation of D-glyceric acid exhibited hyperglycinemia. The opposit inhibition experiment, namely attempts to inhibit the D-glyceric acid metabolism by glycine, was not performed, since the defective enzyme was not known. Accumulation of D-glyceric acid is, however, not seen in the syndrome nonketotic hyperglycinemia, a syndrome that exhibits abnormalities in glycine metabolism very similar to A.J.

There were, however, one feature that neither patients with nonketotic hyperglycinemia nor Durans patient had, namely constant excretion of a number of metabolites derived from accumulated straight-chain and branched-chain acyl-CoA's. This phenomenon was investigated in some detail, since these accumulations might constitute a link between glycine metabolism and D-glyceric acid metabolism.

Both *in vivo* and *in vitro* experiments were performed. These experiments revealed, firstly that the diminution in acyl-CoA degradation rate was located at the level of the acyl-CoA dehydrogenation. Secondly the extent of the diminution was modest compared to what has been found in various inherited defects in the acyl-CoA dehydrogenation. Finally various *in vivo* loading tests seemed to indicate that the diminished rate of acyl-CoA dehydrogenation was secondary to the D-glyceric acid accumulation and possibly due to an endogeneous inhibitor.

Considering the fact, that acyl-CoA's has been implicated in the ethiology of the diminished glycine cleavage activity seen in "ketotic" hyperglycinemia, the following hypothetical sequence of metabolic events in A.J. could then be suggested: 1, a primary defect in the fructose metabolism causing accumulation of a number of compounds including D-glyceric acid; 2, one of these compounds inhibiting the acyl-CoA dehydrogenation causing accumulation of straight-chain and branched-chain acyl-CoA's and excretion of acylglycines; 3, accumulation of acyl-CoA's, which i turn inhibited the glycine cleavage system and thereby caused hyperglycinemia.

An argument against this hypothesis is, however, that the derangement in acyl-CoA metabolism in A.J. seems very modest, compared to what is seen in inborn defects with secundary ("ketotic") hyperglycinemia. Furthermore, the hyperglycinemia in A.J. is of the nonketotic type and not of the "ketotic" type. It should, however, be stated that a few cases of hyperglycinemia of the nonketotic type has been described among patients with propionyl-CoA carboxylase deficiency (Tada *et al.*, 1969; Nishimura *et al.*, 1974; Harris *et al.*,

1981).

Another, and perhaps stronger argument against the proposed metabolic sequence comes from litterature studies. Because the metabolic derangements in A.J. has been characterized in such detail, it has been possible to compare him extensively with those patients from the litterature who excrets similar metabolites.

This comparison has established that A.J., with respect to the D-glyceric acid derangement is comparable with Durans patient, with respect the the glycine derangement is comparable to nonketotic hyperglycinemia and with respect to his deranged acyl-CoA metabolism is at least qualitatively similar to patients with inherited defects in acyl-CoA dehydrogenation. A strong argument against the proposed metabolic sequence is therefore provided by the fact, that Durans patients did not excrete acylglycines in spite of the severe D-glyceric acid accumulation. Similarly, the fact that none of the patients with inherited defects in acyl-CoA dehydrogenation has had hyperglycinemia in spite of high excretion of acylglycines argues against the hypothesis.

Unfortunately the patient died under circumstances where only very limited amounts of liver tissue was secured postmortally. Because of this only cultured fibroblasts were left for further investigations. Since neither the metabolism of fructose, nor the glycine cleavage system is expressed in measurable amounts in this cell type, there are no possibility for further studies into the possible link between glycine and D-glyceric acid.

The total amount of evidence leads therefore, at least for the time being, to the conclusion that A.J. suffered from two different i.e.o.m. at the same time.

6. RESUME

Nærværende oversigtsartikel beskriver samlet de undersøgelser og de overvejelser, der er blevet gjort vedrørende en svært mentalt retarderet dreng, der i 1976 blev fundet i et screening program for i.e.o.m. Drengen udviste et klinisk billede nøje svarende til syndromet nonketotisk hyperglycinemi, nemlig udtalt hypotoni fra få dage efter fødslen, senere efterfulgt af diverse typer kramper og i det senere forløb domineret af svær mental retardering og næsten intraktable kramper. Barnet døde 3 1/2 år gammel i status epilepticus. Ved undersøgelse af urin for ophobede metaboliter fandtes en udtalt accumulation af glycine i mængder svarende til, hvad der findes ved ovennævnte syndrom. Som noget uventet påvistes imidlertid også en svær ophobning af D-glycerinsyre, en metabolit, der på daværende tidspunkt ikke tidligere var set. Herudover påvistes også en, omend mere moderat, ophobning af en række komponenter, der vides at være deriverede fra intracellulært ophobede acyl-CoA'er.

Ved første øjekast ville den mest nærliggende forklaring på dette udskillelsesmønster være, at patienten samtidig havde to forskellige i.e.o.m. Imidlertid er sansynligheden herfor så beskeden at muligheden for en fælles genese til ophobningerne ikke kunne afvises. I forsøget på at klarlægge patientens sygdom blev derfor først de enkelte ophobninger studeret isoleret og sammenlignet med hvad der forelå af informationer i litteraturen om ligenede tilfælde og herefter udførtes en række *in vivo* og *in vitro* forsøg sigtende på at påvise eventuelle forbindelser mellem de forskellige ophobninger.

Hvad angår glycin ophobningen blev det påviste, at fordelingen af glycine mellem blod og cerebrospinal vædsken svarede til hvad der ses i nonketotisk hyperglycinemi, nemlig uforholdmæssig stor accumulation i cerebrospinalvædsken. *In vivo* omsætningsstudier med ^{14}C-l-glycin viste nedsat oxidationshastighed bedømt som produktion af $^{14}CO_2$, et fund, der tyder på en nedsat aktivitet af glycin cleavage systemet, der er den vigtigste nedbrydningvej for glycin. Dette enzym blev derefter målt i postmortelt levervæv fra patienten og fundet nedsat. Transporten af glycin over cellemembranen i dyrkede fibroblaster blev også målt og fundet normal. Disse fund svarer alle nøje til hvad der findes ved syndromet nonketotisk hyperglycinemi.

Hvad angår D-glycerinsyre ophobningen var vanskelighederne større. Initialt måltes enzymet D-glycerate dehydrogenase i leucocyter fra patienten. Der fandtes her en aktivitetsnedsættelse til ca. 25% af normalt. Da imidlertid nedsættelsen syntes for beskeden i forhold til sværhedsgraden af ophobningen, og da der fra litteraturen kendtes et syndrom med umålelig D-glycerat dehydrogenase i kombination med et sygdomsbillede domineret af oxalat udskillelse, udførtes en række *in vivo* loading tests og behandlingsforsøg i et forsøg på mere overordnet at bedømme forstyrrelsen i D-glycerinsyre omsætningen. Disse forsøg viste, at fruktose var precursor for den ophobede D-glycerinsyre. Da den normale fruktose nedbrydning hovedsageligt går via D-glyceraldhyd til 3-fosforglycerate og da den metaboliske pathway fra D-glyceraldehyd til D-glycerinsyre i mennesker synes at ende blindt svarende til D-glycerinsyre, lader disse resultater formode, at defekten må sidde i fruktose stofskiftet i højde med D-glyceraldehyd, og at D-glycerinsyre ophobningen skyldes abnorm shunting ned i den blinde pathway. *In vitro* støtte for en sådan hypothese kunne imidlertid ikke skaffes, da der ikke fandtes tilstrækkeligt lever eller nyre væv til sådanne enzymatiske studier. Efter fundet af den her beskrevne patient er flere andre patienter med D-glycerinsyre ophobning fundet. De to bedst undersøgte af disse har forbavsende nok helt forskellige kliniske billeder og *in vivo* belastninger gav helt modsatte resultater. Den ene af patienterne synes imidlertid både hvad angår klinisk billede og hvad angår belastninger at være helt identisk ned den her beskrevne patient, bortset fra at der ikke findes glycin ophobning.

Hvad angår forsøg på at påvise forbindelse mellem de to ophobninger, blev det i radioaktive tracerstudier vist, at der ikke forekom betydningsfuld omdannelse mellem glycin og D-glycerinsyre *in vivo*. Ligeledes undersøgtes effekten på ophobede metaboliter af dels fruktose belastning, dels behandling med glycin depletering og endelig af riboflavin behandling. I disse forsøg påvistes, at et signifikant fald i glycin udskillelsen, udløst af glycin depletering, ikke påvirkede D-glycerinsyre ophobningen. Modsat resulterede en signifikant stigning i D-glycerinsyre ophobningen, udløst af fruktose, i en noget forsinket og ikke signifikant stigning i glycin udskillelse. Som noget specielt konstateredes samtidig en signifikant stigning i flere af de fra acyl-CoA deriverede metaboliter. Dette sidste var påfaldende, da en række *in vitro* forsøg har indiceret, at netop ophobede acyl-CoA estere skulle have inhiberende effekt på glycin cleavage systemet, og derigennem have betydning for genesen til den hyperglycinemi der ses ved flere i.e.o.m. i de forgrenede aminosyrers nedbrydning. Resultaterne af disse forsøg er forenlige med en hypotese gående ud på at en primær defekt i fruktose stofskifter skulle resultere i en secundær inhibition af acyl-CoA dehydrogeneringen og deraf følgende acyl-CoA ophobning. En eller flere af disse acyl-CoA ester skulle så hæmme glycin cleavage systemet og resultere i hyperglycinemi. Oversigtsartiklen slutter med en række overvejelser over sansynligheden for at en sådan mekanisme skulle spille ind i patientens sygdomsbillede. De data, der foreligger til støtte for hypotesen er alle indirekte. Da samtidig undersøgelserne over genesen til de enkelte ophobninger har godtgjort, at patientens tre metaboliske forstyrrelser hver for sig nøje svarer til, hvad der er fundet i andre patienter, der ikke har denne specielle kombination af ophobninger, må konklusionen intil videre være, at der ikke er nogen forbindelse mellem glycin og D-glycerinsyre forstyrrelsen, og at patienten altså har to uafhængige i.e.o.m. samtidig.

50

REFERENCES

Agamanolis, D.P., Potter, J.L., Herrick, M.K. & Sternberger, N.H. The neuropathology of glycine encephalopathy: A report of five cases with immunohistochemical and ultrastructural observations.
Neurology 32: (1982) 975.

Ando, T., Nyhan, W.L., Gerritsen, T., Gong L., Heiner, D.C. & Bray, P.F. Metabolism of glycine in the nonketotic form of hyperglycinemia.
Pediat. Res. 2: (1968) 254.

Ando, T., Klingenberg, W.G., Ward, A.N., Rasmussen, K. & Nyhan W.L. Isovaleric acidemia presenting with altered metabolism of glycine.
Pediat. Res. 5: (1971 A) 478.

Ando, T. & Nyhan, W.L. The excretion and formation of aminoacetone and δ-aminolevulic acid in man.
Tohoku J. Exp. Med. 99: (1969) 189.

Ando, T., Nyhan, W.L., Connor, J.D., Rasmussen, K., Dommell, K., Barnes, G., Cottem, D. & Hull, D. The oxidation of glycine and propionic acid in propionic acidemia with ketotic hyperglycinemia.
Pediat. Res. 6: (1972) 576.

Ando, T., Rasmussen, R., Nyhan, W.L., Donnell, G.N. & Barnes, N.D. Propionic acidemia in patients with ketotic hyperglycinemia.
J. Pediat. 78 (1971 B) 827.

Aprison, M.H. & Werman, R. The distribution of glycine in cat spinal cord and roots.
Life Sci. 4: (1965) 2075.

Applegarth, D.A. & Poon, S. Interpretation of elevated blood glycine levels in children.
Clin. Chim. Acta 63: (1975) 49.

Arnstein, H.R.V. & Neuberger, A. The synthesis of glycine and serine by the rat.
Biochem. J. 55: (1953) 271.

Balcar, V.J. & Johnston, G.A.R. High affinity uptake of transmitters: Studies on the uptake of L-aspartate, GABA, L-glutamate and glycine in cat spinal cord.
J. Neurochem. 20: (1973) 529.

Banks, W.J.& Morrow, G. A familial spinal cord disorder with hyperglycinemia.
Arch. Neurol. 27: (1972) 136.

Bartlett, K. & Gompertz, D. The specificity of glycine-N-acylase and acylglycine excretion in the organic acidemias.
Biochem. Med. 10: (1974) 15.

Baumgartner, R., Ando, T. & Nyhan, W.L. Nonketotic hyperglycinemia.
J. Pediat. 75: (1969) 1022.

Beinert, H. Acyl-coenzyme A dehydrogenases. In Boyer, P.D., Lardy, H. & Myrback, K. (eds.) The enzymes. 2nd ed.
Academic Press, New York, 1963. p 447.

Berger, S.J., Carter, J.G. & Lowry, O.H. The distribution of glycine, GABA, glutamate and aspartate in rabbit spinal cord, cerebellum and hippocampus.
J. Neurochem. 28: (1977) 149.

Bernardina, B.D., Aicardi, J., Goutieres, F. & Plouin, P. Glycine encephalopathy.
Neuropädiatrie 10: (1979) 209.

Bito, L., Dawson, H., Levin, E., Murray, M. & Snider, N. The concentrations of free amino acids and other electrolytes in cerebrospinal fluid, in vivo dialysate of brain, and blood plasma of the dog.
J. Neurochem. 13: (1966) 1057.

Bradford, H.F., Bennett, G.W. & Thomas, A.J. Depolarizing stimuli and the release of physiologically active amino acids from suspensions of mammalian synaptosomes.
J. Neurochem. 21: (1973) 495.

Brandt, N.J., Brandt, S., Rasmussen K & Schønheyder, F. Hyperglyceric-acidemia with hyperglycinemia: a new inborn error of metabolism.
Br. Med. J. 4: (1974) 344.

Brandt, N.J., Rasmussen, K., Brandt, S., Kølvraa, S. & Schønheyder, F. D-glyceric acidemia and non-ketotic hyperglycinemia.
Acta Pædiatr. Scand. 65: (1976) 17.

Bridgers, W.F. The biosynthesis of serine in mouse brain extracts.
J. Biol. Chem. 240: (1965) 4591.

Bruin, W.J., Frantz, B.M. & Sallach, H.J. The occurrence of a glycine cleavage system in mammalian brain.
J. Neurochem. 20: (1973) 1649.

Brun, A., Börjeson, M., Hultberg, B., Sjöblad, S., Akesson, H. & Litwin, E. Neonatal non-ketotic hyperglycinemia: A clinical, biochemical and neuropathological study including electronmicroscopic findings.
Neuropädiatrie 10: (1979) 195.

Carson, N.A.J. Non-ketotic hyperglycinemia: A review of 70 patients.
J. Inher. Metab. Dis. 5: (1982) 126.

Caldwell, J., Moffatt, J.R. & Smith, R.L. Post-mortem survival of hippuric acid formation in rat and human cadaver tissue samples.
Xenobiotica 6: (1976) 275.

Cherruau, B., Mangeot, M., Demelier, J.F., Charpentier, C., Pelletier, C. & Lemonnier, A. Metabolic abnormalities observed in the rat after administration of sodium dipropylacetate.
Toxic. Lett. 8: (1981) 39.

Cheung, G.P., Cotropia, J.P. & Sallach, H.J. The effects of diatary protein on the hepatic enzymes of serine metabolism in the rabbit.
Arch. Biochem. Biophys 129: (1969) 672.

Childs, B., Nyhan, W.L., Borden, M., Bard, L. & Cooke, R.E. Idiopathic hyperglycinemia and hyperglycinuria: A new disorder of amino acid metabolism. I.
Pediatrics 27: (1961) 522.

Cochrane, W., Scriver, C.R. & Krause, V. Hyperglycinemia-hyperglycinuria syndrome in a newborn infant. Abstract.
Soc. Pediat. Res. Atlantic City (1963). p 102.

Coderch, R., Luis, C. & Bozal, J. Effects of salts on D-glycerate dehydrogenase kinetic behavior.
Biochim. Biophys. Acta 566: (1979) 21.

Coulter, D.L. and Allen, R.J. Hyperammonemia with valproic acid therapy.
J. Pediat. 99: (1981) 317.

Christensen, E., Jacobsen, B.B., Gregersen, N., Hjeds, H., Pedersen, J.B., Brandt, N.J. & Baekmark, U.B. Urinary excretion of succinylacetone and δ-aminolevulinic acid in patients with hereditary tyrosinemia.
Clin. Chim. Acta. 116 (1981) 331.

Christensen, E., Kølvraa, S. & Gregersen, N. Glutaric aciduria type II: Evidence for a defect related to the electron transfer flavoprotein or its dehydrogenase.
Pediat. Res. 18: (1984) 663.

Christensen, H.N. Biological transport.
Benjamin Reading, New York 1975, p. 174.

Curtis, D.R., Game, C.J.A. & Lodge, D. Benzodiazepines and central glycine receptors.
Br. J. Pharmac. 56: (1976) 307.

Curtis, D.R. Hösli, L., Johnston, G.A.R. & Johnston, I.H. The hyperpolarization of spinal motoneurones by glycine and related amino acids.
Exp. Brain Res. 5: (1968 A) 235.

Curtis, D.R., Hösli, L. & Johnston, G.A.R. A pharmacological study of the depression of spinal neurones by glycine and related amino acids.
Exp. Brain Res. 6: (1968 B) 1.

Cutler, R.W.P., Murray, J.E. & Hammerstad, J. P. Role of mediated transport in the electrically-induced release of (^{14}C)glycine from slices of rat spinal cord.
J. Neurochem. 19: (1972) 539.

Daly, E.C. & Aprison, M.H. Distribution of serine hydroxymethyltransferase and glycine transaminase in several areas of the central nervous system of the rat.
J. Neurochem 22: (1974) 877.

Daly, E.C., Nadi, N.S. & Aprison, M.H. Regional distribution and properties of the glycine cleavage system within the central nervous system of the rat: evidence for an endogeneous inhibitor during *in vitro* assay.
J. Neurochem. 26: (1976) 179.

Daum, R.S., Scriver, C.R., Mamer, O.A., Delvin, E., Lamm, P. & Goldman, H. An inherited disorder of isoleucine catabolism causing accumulation of α-methylacetoacetate and α-methyl-β-hydroxybutyrate, and intermittent metabolic acidosis.
Pediat. Res. 7: (1973) 149.

Davidoff, R.A. & Adair, R. High affinity amino acid transport by frog spinal cord slices.
J. Neurochem 24: (1975) 545.

Davidoff, R.A. & Adair, R. GABA and glycine transport in frog CNS: High affinity uptake and potassium-evoked release *in vitro*.
Brain Res. 118: (1976) 403.

Davies, L.P. & Johnston, G.A.R. Serine hydroxymethyl transferase in the central nervous system: Regional and subcellular distribution studies.
Brain Res. 54: (1973) 149.

Davies, L.P. & Johnston, G.A.R. Postnatal changes in the levels of glycine and the activities of serine hydroxymethyltransferase and glycine: 2-oxoglutarate aminotransferase in the rat central nervous system.
J. Neurochem. 22: (1974) 107.

Dawkins, P.D. & Dickens, F. The oxidation of D- and L-glycerate by rat liver.
Biochem. J. 94: (1965) 353.

de Groot, C.J., Everts, V.B., Touwen, B.C.L. & Hommes, F.A. Non-ketotic hyperglycinemia: An inborn error of metabolism affecting brain function exclusively.
Prog. Brain Res. 48: (1978) 199.

de Groot, C.J., Touwen, B.C.L., Huisjes, H.J. & Hommes, F.A. Early findings of a case of non-ketotic hyperglycinemia.
Ann. Clin. Biochem. 14: (1977) 140.

de Groot, G.J., Troelstra, J.A. & Hommes, F.A. Non-ketotic hyperglycinemia: an *in vitro* study of the glycine-serine conversion in liver of three patients and the effect of dietary methionine.
Pediat. Res. 4: (1970) 238.

Dixon, M. & Kleppe, K. D-amino acid oxidase. Specificity, competitive inhibition, and reaction sequence.
Biochim. Biophys. Acta 96: (1965) 368.

Dudzinski, D.S. & Cutler, R.W.P. Spinal subarachnoid perfusion in the rat: glycine transport from spinal fluid.
J. Neurochem. 22: (1974) 355.

Duran, M., Beemer, F.A., Bruinvis, L., Ketting, D. and Wadman, S.K. D-glyceric acidemia: An inborn error associated with fructose metabolism.
Ped. Res. 1988, (in press).

Duran, M., Ketting, D., Dorland, L. and Wadman, S.K. The identification of acylcarnitines by desorption chemical ionization mass spectrometry.
J. Inher. Metab. Dis. 8 suppl 2 (1985) 143.

Ehinger, B. & Lindberg-Bauer, B. Light-evoked release of glycine from cat and rabbit retina.
Brain Res. 113: (1976) 535.

Ewlyn, D., Ashmore, J., Cahill, G.F. Zotty, S., Welch, W. & Hastings, A.B. Serine metabolism in rat liver slices.
J. Biol. Chem. 226: (1957) 735.

Fallon, H.J., Hackney, E.J. & Byrne, W.L. Serine biosynthesis in rat liver.
J. Biol. Chem. 241: (1966) 4157.

Fernhoff, P.M. Ahmann, P.A. & Elsas, L.J. Renal tubular transport of amino acids in non-ketotic hyperglycinemia: Effects of valine restriction and strychnine therapy.
Pediat. Res. 12: (1978) 812A.

Flannery, D.B., Pellock, J., Bousounis, D., Hunt, P., Nance, C. & Wolf, B. Nonketotic hyperglycinemia in two retarded adults: A mild form of infantile nonketotic hyperglycinemia.
Neurology 33: (1983) 1064.

Forman, W.B., Davidson, E.D. & Webster, L.T. Enzymatic conversion of salicylate to salicylurate.
Molecular Pharmacology 7: (1971) 247.

Frereman, F.E. & Goodman, S.I. Deficiency of electron transfer flavoprotein or electron transfer flavoprotein ubiquinone oxidoreductase in glutaric acidemia Type II fibroblasts.
Proc. Natl, Acad. Sci. (USA) 82: (1985) 4517.

Fujiwara, K., Okamura, K. & Motokawa, Y. Hydrogen carrier protein from chicken liver: purification, characterization and role of its prosthetic group, lipoic acid, in the glycine cleavage reaction.
Arch. Biochem. Biophys. 197: (1979) 454.

Gatley, S.J. & Sherratt, H.S.A. The synthesis of hippurate from benzoate and glycine by rat liver mitochondria.
Biochem. J. 166: (1977) 39.

Gerritsen, T., Kaveggia, E. & Waisman, H.A. A new type of idiopatic hyperglycinemia with hyperoxaluria.
Pediatrics 36: (1965) 882.

Gitzelmann, R., Steinmann, B. Otten, A., Dumermuth, G., Herdan, M., Reubi, J.C. & Cuenod, M. Nonketotic hyperglycinemia treated with strychnine, a glycine receptor antagonist.
Helv. Pediat. Acta 32: (1977) 517.

Gold, M.R. & Martin, A.R. Analysis of glycine-activated inhibitory post-synaptic channels in brain-stem neurones of the lamprey.
J. Physiol. 342: (1983) 99.

Gold, M.R. & Martin, A.R. γ-aminobutyric acid and glycine activate Cl⁻ channels having different characteristics in CNS neurones.
Nature 308: (1984) 639.

Gompertz, D., Bau, D.C.K., Storrs, C.N., Peters, T.J. & Hughes, E.A. Localization of enzymatic defect in propionic acidemia.
Lancet 1: (1970) 1140.

Gompertz, D., Saudubray, J.M., Charpentier, C., Bartlett, K., Goodey, P.A., & Draffan, G.H. A defect in L-isoleucine metabolism associated with α-methyl-β-hydroxybutyric acid and α-methylacetoacetic aciduria: quantitative *in vivo* and *in vitro* studies.
Clin. Chim. Acta 57: (1974) 269.

Grandgeorge, M.D. L'acidemie D. glycerique. Anormalie hereditaire du metabolisme de la glycine.
These. Universite scientifique et medicale de Grenoble, 1979.

Gravel, R.A., Lam, K.F., Scully, K.J. & Hsia, Y.E. Genetic complementation of propionyl-CoA carboxylase deficiency in cultured human fibroblasts.
Am. J. Hum. Genet. 29: (1977) 378.

Green, R.C. & Radovich, C. Role of methionine in the regulation of serine hydroxymethyltransferase in *Escherichia coli*.
J. Bact. 124: (1975) 269.

Gregersen, N. The acyl-CoA dehydrogenation deficiencies.
Scand. J. Clin. Invest. 45, suppl. 174: (1985) 1.

Gregersen, N., Kølvraa, S., Rasmussen, K., Mortensen, P.B., Divry, P., David, M. & Hobolth, N. General (medium chain) acyl-CoA dehydrogenase deficiency (non-ketotic dicarboxylic aciduria): Quantitative urinary excretion pattern of 23 biologically significant organic acids in three cases.
Clin. Chim. Acta 132: (1983) 181.

Gregersen, N., Kølvraa, S. & Mortensen, P.B. Acyl-CoA: glycine acyltransferase: *on vitro* studies on the glycine conjugation of straight- and branched-chained acyl-CoA's in human liver.
Biochem. Med. and Metab. Biol. 35: (1986) 210.

Gregersen, N., Lauritzen, R. & Rasmussen, K. Suberylglycine excretion in the urine from a patient with dicarboxylic aciduria
Clin. Chim. Acta 70: (1976) 417.

Gregersen, N., Wintzensen, H., Kølvraa, S., Christensen, E., Christensen, M.F., Brandt, N.J. & Rasmussen, K. C_6-C_{10}-dicarboxylic aciduria: Investigations of a patient with riboflavin responsive multiple acyl-CoA dehydrogenation defects.
Pediat. Res. 16: (1982) 861.

Guynn, R.W. Equilibrium constants under physiological conditions for the reactions of the nonphosphorylated pathway of serine biosynthesis.
Arch. Biochem. Biophys. 218: (1982) 14.

Hale, D.E., Batshaw, M.L., Coates, P.M., Frerman, F.E., Goodman, S.I., Singh, I. & Stanley, C.A. Long-chain acyl-CoA dehydrogenase deficiency: An inherited cause of nonketotic hypoglycemia.
Pediat. Res. 19: (1985) 666.

Hall, C.L. Electron-transfer flavoprotein from pig liver mitochondria.
Methods Enzymol. 71: (1981) 386.

Halton, D.M. & Krieger, I. Studies of glycine metabolism and transport in fibroblasts from patients with nonketotic hyperglycinemia.
Pediat. Res. 14: (1980) 932.

Hampton, R.K., Barron, L.L. & Olson, M.S. Regulation of the glycine cleavage system in isolated rat liver mitochondria.
J. Biol. Chem. 258: (1983) 2993.

Hampton, R.K., Taylor, M.K. & Olson, M. S. Regulation of the glycine cleavage system in isolated perfused rat liver.
J. Biol. Chem. 259: (1984) 1180.

Harris, D.J., Thompson, R.M., Wolf, B. & Yang, B.I. Propionyl coenzyme A carboxylase deficiency presenting as non-ketotic hyperglycinemia.
J. Med. Genet. 18: (1981) 156.

Hayasaka, K., Kochi, H., Hiraga, K. & Kikuchi, G. Purification and properties of glycine decarboxylase, a component of the glycine cleavage system, from rat liver mitochondria and immunochemical comparison of this enzyme from various sources.
J. Biochem. 88: (1980) 1193.

Hayasaka, K., Narisawa, K., Satoh. T., Tateda, H., Metoki, K., Tada, K., Hiraga, K., Aoki, T., Kawakami, T., Akamatsu, H. & Matsuo, N. Glycine cleavage system in ketotic hyperglycinemia: a reduction of H-protein activity.
Pediat. Res. 16: (1982) 5.

Hayasaka, K. & Tada, K. Effects of metabolites of the branched-chain amino acids and cysteamine on the glycine cleavage system.
Biochem. Intern. 6: (1983) 225.

Hayasaka, K., Tada, K., Kikuchi, G., Winter, S. & Nyhan, W.L. Nonketotic hyperglycinemia: Two patients with primary defects of P-protein and T-protein, respectively, in the glycine cleavage system.
Pediat. Res. 17: (1983) 967.

Heinz, F. Metabolism of fructose in liver.
Acta Med. Scand. Suppl. 542: (1972) 27.

Heinz, F., Lamprecht, W. & Kirsch, J. Enzymes of fructose metabolism in human liver.
J. Clin. Invest. 47: (1968) 1826.

Hillman, R. E. & Otto, E.F. Inhibition of glycine-serine interconversion in cultured human fibroblasts by products of isoleucine catabolism.
Pediat. Res. 8: (1974) 941.

Hillman. R.E., Sowers, L.H. & Cohen, J.L. Inhibition of glycine oxidation in cultured fibroblasts by isoleucine.
Pediat. Res. 7: (1973) 945.

Hiraga, K. & Kikuchi, G. The mitochondrial glycine cleavage system. Purification & properties of glycine decarboxylase from chicken liver mitochondria.
J. Biol. Chem. 255: (1980 A) 11664.

Hiraga, K. & Kikuchi, G. The mitochondrial glycine cleavage system. Functional association of glycine decarboxylase and aminomethyl carrier protein.
J. Biol. Chem. 255: (1980 B) 11671.

Hiraga, K., Kochi, H., Hayasaka, K., Kikuchi, G. & Nyhan, W.L. Defective glycine cleavage system in nonketotic hyperglycinemia.
J. Clin. Invest. 68: (1981) 525.

Hommes, F.A., Kuipers, J.R.G., Elema, J.D., Jansen, J.F. & Jonxis, J.H. P. Propionic acidemia, a new inborn error of metabolism.
Pediat. Res. 2: (1968) 519.

Hsia, Y.E., Scully, K.J. & Rosenberg, L.E. Defective propionate carboxylation in ketotic hyperglycinemia.
Lancet 1: (1969) 757.

Hsia. Y.E. Scully, K.J. & Rosenberg, L.E. Inherited propionyl-CoA carboxylase deficiency in "ketotic hyperglycinemia"
J. Clin. Invest. 50: (1971) 127.

Hue, L. & Hers, H. G. The conversion of (4-^{3}H) fructose and of (4-^{3}H) glucose to liver glycogen in the mouse.
Eur. J. Biochem. 29: (1972) 268.

Hökfelt, T. & Ljungdahl, Å. Light and electron microscopic autoradiography on spinal cord slices after incubation with labelled glycine.
Brain Res. 32: (1971) 189.

Ichihara, A & Greenberg D.M. Studies on the purification and properties of D-glyceric acid kinase of liver.
J. Biol. Chem. 225: (1957) 949.

Ikeda, Y., Okamura-Ikeda, K. and Tanaka, K. Purification and characterization of short-chain, medium-chain and long-chain acyl-CoA dehydrogenases from rat liver mitochondria.
J. Biol. Chem. 260: (1985) 1311.

Ikeda, Y. & Tanaka, K. Isolation of 2-Me-branched-chain acyl-CoA dehydrogenase from rat liver mitochondria.
Fed.Proc. 41: (1982) 1192.

Ikeda, Y. & Tanaka, K. Purification and characterization of isovaleryl coenzyme A dehydrogenase from rat liver mitochondria.
J. Biol.Chem. 258: (1983) 1077.

Jaeken, J., Corbeel, L., Casaer, P., Carchon, H., Eggermont, E. and Eeckels, R. Dipropylacetate (valproate) and glycine metabolism.
Lancet 2: (1977) 617.

James, M.O. & Bend, J. R. Perinatal developement of, and effect of chemical pretreatment on, glycine N-acyltransferase activities in liver and kidney of rabbit and rat.
Biochem. J. 172: (1978) 293.

James, M.O., Smith, R.L., Williams, R.T. & Reidenberg, M. The conjugation of phenylacetic acid in man, subman primates and some non-primate species.
Proc. R. Soc. Lond. B. 182: (1972) 25.

Johnston, G.A.R. & Iversen, L.L. Glycine uptake in rat central nervous system slices and homogenate: Evidence for different uptake systems in spinal cord and cerebral cortex.
J. Neurochem. 18: (1971) 1951.

Kattermann, R., Dold, U. & Holzer, H. D-glycerat beim fructoseabbau in der leber.
Biochemische Zeitschrift 334: (1961) 218.

Keating, J.P., Feigin, R.D., Tenenbaum, S.M. & Hillman, R.E. Hyperglycinemia with ketosis due to a defect in isoleucine metabolism: a preliminary report.
Pediatr. 50: (1972) 890.

Kelly, J.C., Otto, E.F. & Hillman, R.E. Glycine transport by human diploid fibroblasts. Absence of a defect in cells from patients with nonketotic hyperglycinemia.
Pediat. Res. 13: (1979) 127.

Kikuchi, G. The glycine cleavage system: Composition, reaction mechanism and physiological significance.
Mol. Cell. Biochem. 1: (1973) 169.

Kikuchi, G. & Hiraga, K. The mitochondrial glycine cleavage system.
Mol. Cell. Biochem. 45: (1982) 137.

Kikuchi, G., Hiraga, K. & Yoshida, T. Role of the glycine cleavage system in glycine and serine metabolism in various organs.
Biochem. Soc. Trans. 8: (1980) 504.

Kitagawa, Y., Katayama, H. & Sugimoto, E. Identity of mitochondrial and cytosolic glycerate kinases in rat liver and regulation of their intracellular localisation by dietary protein.
Biochim. Biophys. Acta 582: (1979) 260.

Kitagawa, Y. & Sugimoto, E. Possibility of mitochondrial-cytosolic cooperation in glyconeogenesis from serine via hydroxypyruvate.
Biochim. Biophys. Acta 582: (1979) 276.

Kitagawa, Y., Sugimoto, E. & Chiba, H. Regulatory properties of beef liver D-glycerate dehydrogenase.
Agr. Biol. Chem. 39: (1975A) 193.

Kitagawa, Y., Sugimoto, E. & Chiba, H. Subunits and sulfhydryl groups of beef liver D-glycerate dehydrogenase.
Agr. Biol. Chem. 39: (1975B) 199.

Kochi, H., Hayasaka, K., Hiraga, K. & Kikuchi, G. Reduction of the level of the glycine cleavage system in the rat liver resulting from administration of dipropylacetate.
Arch. Biochem. Biophys. 198: (1979) 589.

Kontro, P., Marnela, K.M. & Oja, S.S. Free amino acids on the synaptosomes and synaptic vesicle fractions of different bovine brain areas.
Brain Res. 184: (1980) 129.

Kretchmar, A.L. & Price, E.J. Use of respiration pattern analysis for study of serine metabolism *in vivo*.
Metabolism 18: (1969) 684.

Krieger, I. & Tanaka, K. Therapeutic effects of glycine in isovaleric acidemia.
Pediat. Res. 10: (1976) 25.

Krieger, I., Winbaum, E.S. & Eisenbrey, A.B. Cerebrospinal fluid glycine in nonketotic hyperglycinemia. Effect of treatment with sodium benzoate and a ventricular shunt.
Metabolism. 26: (1977) 517.

Kølvraa, S. Inhibition of the glycine cleavage system by branched-chain amino acid metabolites.
Pediat. Res. 13: (1979) 889.

Kølvraa, S., Brandt, N.J. & Christensen, E. Nonketotic hyperglycinemia. Clinical, biochemical and therapeutic aspects.
Acta. Paed. Scand. 68: (1979) 629.

Kølvraa, S., Christensen, E. & Brandt, N.J. Studies of the glycine metabolism in a patient with D-glyceric acidemia and hyperglycinemia.
Pediat. Res. 14: (1980B) 1029.

Kølvraa, S. & Gregersen, N. Acyl-CoA: glycine acyltransferase: Organelle localisation and affinity towards straight- and branched-chained acyl-CoA's in rat liver.
Biochem. Med. and Metab. Biol. 36: (1986) 105.

Kølvraa, S., Gregersen, N. & Brandt. N.J. Excretion of short-chain N-acylglycines in the urine of a patient with D-glyceric acidemia.
Clin. Chim. Acta 106: (1980A) 215.

Kølvraa, S., Gregersen, N. & Christensen, E. *In vivo* studies on the metabolic derangement in a patient with D-glyceric acidemia and hyperglycinemia.
J. Inher. Metab. Dis. 7: (1984) 49.

Kølvraa, S., Gregersen, N., Christensen, E. & Hobolth, N. *In vitro* fibroblast studies in a patient with C_6-C_{10}-dicarboxylic aciduria: Evidence for a defect in general acyl-CoA dehydrogenase.
Clin. Chim. Acta 126: (1982) 53.

Kølvraa, S., Rasmussen, K. & Brandt, N.J. D-glyceric acidemia: Biochemical studies of a new syndrome.
Pediat. Res. 10: (1976) 825.

Kølvraa, S., Rosleff, F. & Brandt, N.J. Normal glycine transport in cultured diploid fibroblasts from hyperglycinemic subjects.
J. Inher. Metab. Dis. 6: (1983) 82.

Lau, E. P., Haley, B.E. & Barden, R.E. Photoaffinity labelling of acyl-CoA.:glycine N-acyltransferase with p-azidobenzoyl-CoA.
Biochemistry 16: (1977) 2581.

Leupold, D., Przyrembel, H., Heymer, D., Hilgarth, R., Krüger, C., Peiffer, J. & Bremer, H.J. Nichtketotische hyperglycinämie.
Z. Kinder Heilk. 116: (1974) 95.

Liao, L.L. & Richardson, K.E. The synthesis of oxalate from hydroxypyruvate by isolated perfused rat liver.
Biochim. Biophys. Acta 538: (1978) 76.

Logan, W.L. & Snyder, S.H. High-affinity uptake system for glycine, glutamic and aspartic acids in synaptosomes of rat cerebral nervous tissue Brain Res. 42: (1972) 413.

Mabry, C.C. & Karam, A. Idiopathic hyperglycinemia & hyperglycinuria.
Southern Med. J. 56: (1963) 1444.

MacDermot, K.D., Nelson, W., Reichert, C.M. & Schulman, J.D. Attempts at use of strychnine sulfate in the treatment of non-ketotic hyperglycinemia.
Pediatr. 65: (1980) 61.

Mantagos, S., Genel, M. & Tanaka, K. Ethylmalonic-adipic aciduria. In vivo and in vitro studies indicating deficiency of activities of multiple acyl-CoA dehydrogenases.
J. Clin. Invest. 64: (1979) 1580.

Matalon, R., Naidu, S., Hughes, J.R. & Michals, K. Nonketotic hyperglycinemia: Treatment with diazepam. A competitor for glycine receptors.
Pediatr. 71: (1983) 581.

McBride, W.J., Daly, E. & Aprison, M.H. Interconversion of glycine and serine in a synaptosome fraction isolated from the spinal cord, medulla oblongata, telencephalon, and cerebellum of the rat.
J. Neurobiol. 4: (1973) 557.

McKeon, C., Eanes, R.Z., Fall, R.R., Tasset, D.M. & Wolf, B. Immunological studies of propionyl-CoA carboxylase in livers and fibroblasts of patients with propionic acidemia.
Clin. Chim. Acta 101: (1980) 217.

Meedel, T.H. & Pizer, L.I. Regulation of one-carbon biosynthesis and utilization in *Escherichia coli*.
J. Bact. 118: (1974) 905.

Miyata, Y. & Otsuka, M. Quantitative histochemistry of γ-aminobutyric acid in cat spinal cord with special reference to presynaptic inhibition.
J. Neurochem. 25: (1975) 239.

Mortensen, P.B., Kølvraa, S. & Christensen, E. Inhibition of the glycine cleavage system: Hyperglycinemia and hyperglycinuria caused by valproic acid.
Epilepsia 21: (1980) 563.

Motokawa, Y. & Kikuchi, G. Glycine metabolism in rat liver mitochondria. Intramitochondrial localization of the reversible glycine cleavage system and serine hydroxymethyltransferase. Arch.
Biochem. Biophys. 146: (1971) 461.

Motokawa, Y. & Kikuchi, G. Glycine metabolism by rat liver mitochondria.
Arch. Biochem. Biophys. 164: (1974) 624.

Murray, J.E. & Cutler, R.W.P. Clearance of glycine from cat cerebrospinal fluid: faster clearance from spinal subarachnoid than from ventricular compartment.
J. Neurochem. 17: (1970) 703.

Nakano, Y., Fujika, M. & Wada, H. Studies on serine hydroxymethyltransferase isoenzymes from rat liver.
Biochim. Biophys. Acta 159: (1968) 19.

Nandi, D.L., Lucas. S.V. & Webster, L.T. Benzoyl-CoA: glycine N-acyltransferase and phenylacetyl-CoA: glycine N-acyltransferase from bovine liver mitochondria: purification and characterization.
J. Biol. Chem. 254: (1979) 7230.

Nishimura, Y., Tada, K. & Arakawa, T. Coexistence of defective activity in glycine cleavage reaction and propionyl-CoA carboxylase in the liver of a hyperglycinemic child.
Tohoku J. Exp. Med. 113: (1974) 267.

Nyhan, W.L., Ando, T. And Rasmussen, K. Ketotic hyperglycinemia. in Stern, J. and Toothill, C., (eds.): Organic acidurias.
Churchill Livingstone, London 1972. p 1.

Nyhan, W. L., Borden, M. & Childs, B. Idiopathic hyperglycinemia: A new disorder of amino acid metabolism.
Pediatr. 27: (1961) 539.

Nyhan, W.L. & Childs, B. Hyperglycinemia V. The miscible pool and turnover rate of glycine and the formation of serine.
J. Clin. Invest. 43: (1964) 2404.

Nyhan, W.L., Chisolm, J.J. & Edwards, R.O. Idiopathic hyperglycinuria.
J. Pediatr. 62:; (1963) 540.

Oberholzer, V.G., Levin. B. Burgess, E.A. & Young, W.F. Methylmalonic aciduria. An inborn error of metabolism leading to chronic metabolic acidosis.
Arch. Dis. Childh. 42: (1967) 492.

O'Brien, W. Inhibition of glycine synthase by branched-chain α-keto acids.
Arch. Biochem. Biophys. 189: (1978) 291.

Ogawa, H. & Fujika, M. Purification and characterization of cytosolic and mitochondrial serine hydroxymethyltransferases from rat liver.
J. Biochem (Tokyo) 90: (1981) 381.

Okamura-Ikeda, K., Fujiwara, K. & Motokawa, Y. Purification and characterization of chicken liver T-protein, a compound of the glycine cleavage system.
J. Biol. Chem. 257: (1982) 135.

Oldendorf, W.H. Brain uptake of radiolabelled amino acids, amines, and hexoses after arterial injection.
Am. J. Physiol. 6: (1971) 1629.

Osmundsen, H. & Bremer, J. A spectrophotometric procedure for rapid and sensitive measurements of β-oxidation.
Biochem. J. 164: (1977) 621.

Patrick, J.T., McBride, W.J. & Felten, D.L. Distribution of glycine, GABA, aspartate and glutamate in the rat spinal cord.
Brain Res. Bull. 10: (1983) 415.

Perry, T.L., Urquhart, N., Hansen, S. & Mamer, O.A. Studies of the glycine cleavage enzyme system in brains from infants with glycine encephalopathy.
Pediat. Res. 12: (1977) 1192.

Perry, T.L., Urquhart, N., MacLean, J., Evans, M.E., Hansen, S., Davidson, A.G.F., Applegarth, D.A., MacLeod, P.J. & Lock, J.E. Nonketotic hyperglycinemia: glycine accumulation due to absence of glycine cleavage in brain.
N. Engl. J. Med. 292: (1975) 1269.

Pollay, M. Movement of glycine across the blood-brain barrier of the rabbit.
J. Neurobiol. 7: (1975) 123.

Price, C.H. & McAdoo, D.J. Localization of axonally transported (^{3}H) glycine in vesicles of identified neurones.
Brain Res. 219: (1981) 307.

Raghavan, K.G. & Richardson, K.E. Hyperoxaluria in L-glyceric aciduria: Possible nonenzymatic mechanism.
Biochem. Med. 29: (1983) 114.

Ramesh, K.S. & Rao, N.A. Purification and physicochemical, kinetic and immunological properties of allosteric serine hydroxymethyltransferase from monkey liver.
Biochem. J. 187: (1980) 623.

Rampini, S., Vischer, D., Curtius, H.C., Anders, P.W., Tancredi, F., Frischknecht, W. & Prader, A. Heriditäre Hyperglycinämie.
Helv. Paediet. Acta 22: (1967) 135.

Ratner, S., Nocito, V. & Green, D.E. Glycine oxidase.
J. Biol. Chem. 152: (1944) 119.

Ratner, S., Ritterberg, D., Keston, A.S. & Schoenheimer, R. Studies in protein metabolism.
J. Biol. Chem. 134: (1940) 665.

Revsin, B. & Morrow, G. Glycine transport in normal and non-ketotic hyperglycinemic human diploid fibroblasts.
Exp. Cell Res. 100: (1976) 95.

Rhead, W., Hall, C.L. & Tanaka, K. Novel tritium release assays for isovaleryl-CoA and butyryl-CoA dehydrogenases.
J. Biol. Chem. 256: (1981) 1616.

Rhead, W.J. & Tanaka, K. Demonstration of a specific mitochondrial isovaleryl-CoA dehydrogenase deficiency in fibroblasts from patients with isovaleric acidemia.
Proc. Natl. Acad. Sci. USA. 77: (1980) 580.

Roberts, P.J. & Mitchell, J.F. The release of amino acids from the hemisected spinal cord during stimulation.
J. Neurochem. 19: (1972) 2473.

Rosenberg, L.E. Disorders of Propionate and methylmalonate metabolism. in Stanbury, J.B., Wyngaarden, J.G., Fredrickson, D.S., Goldstein, J.L. & Brown, M.S., (eds.): The metabolic basis of inherited disease.
McGraw-Hill Book Co. New York 1983. p 474.

66

Rosenberg, L.E. & Scriver, R.C. Disorders of glycine metabolism. in Bondy, P.K. & Rosenberg, L.E., (eds.).: Metabolic control and disease.
W.B. Saunders Co., Philadelphia, 1980. p 672.

Rosenblum, I.Y., Antkowiak, D.H., Sallach, H.J., Flanders, L.E. & Fahien, L.A. Purification and regulatory properties of beef liver D-glycerate dehydrogenase.
Arch. Biochem. Biophys. 144: (1971) 375.

Rowsell, E.V., Al-Naama, M.M. & Rowsell, K.V. Glycine metabolism in rat kidney cortex slices.
Biochem. J. 204: (1982) 313.

Rowsell, E.V., Snell, K., Carnie, J.A. & Al-Tai, A.H. Liver L-alanine-glyoxylate and L-serine-pyruvate aminotransferase activities: An apparent association with gluconeogenesis.
Biochem. J. 115: (1969) 1071.

Ruzicka, F.J. & Beinert, H. A new ion-sulfur flavoprotein of the respiratory chain.
J. Biol. Chem. 252: (1977) 8440.

Sakami, W. The conversion of formate and glycine to serine and glycogen in the intact rat.
J. Biol. Chem. 176: (1948) 995.

Sakami, W. The conversion of glycine into serine in the intact rat.
J. Biol. Chem. 178: (1949) 519.

Sato, T., Kochi, H., Motokawa, Y., Kawasaki, H. & Kikuchi, G. Glycine metabolism by rat liver mitochondria.
J. Biochem. 65: (1969 A) 63.

Sato, T., Kochi, H., Sata, N. & Kikuchi, G. Glycine metabolism by rat liver mitochondria.
J. Biochem. 65: (1969 B) 77.

Saudubray, J.M., Sorin, M., Depondt, E., Herouin, C., Charpentier, C. & Pousset, J.L. Acidemie isovalerique. Etude et traitement chez trois freres.
Arch. Franc. Ped. 33: (1976) 795.

Schachter, D. & Taggart, J.V. Benzoyl coenzyme A and hippurate synthesis.
J. Biol. Chem. 203: (1953) 925.

Schreier, V.K. & Müller, W. Idiopathische Hyperglycinämie (Glycinose).
Dtsch. Med. Wschr. 89: (1964) 1739.

Sestoft, L., Damgaard, S., Tygstrup, N. & Lundquist, F. Metabolism of fructose and glyceraldehyde in isolated perfused pig liver.
Acta Med. Scand. Suppl. 542: (1972) 119.

Shank, R.P. & Aprison, M.H. The metabolism *in vivo* of glycine and serine in eight areas of the rat central nervous system.
J. Neurochem. 17: (1970) 1461.

Shank, R.P., Aprison, M.H. & Baxter, C.F. Precursors of glycine in the nervous system: comparison of specific activities in glycine and other amino acids after administration of (U-^{14}C) glucose, (3,4-^{14}C) glucose, (1-^{14}C) glucose, (U-^{14}C) serine or (1,5-^{14}C) citrate to the rat.
Brain Res. 52: (1973) 301.

Sillero, M.A.G., Sillero, A. & Sols, A. Enzymes involved in fructose metabolism in liver and the glyceraldehyde metabolic crossroads.
Eur. J. Biochem. 10: (1969) 345.

Similä, S. & Visakorpi, J.K. Clinical findings in three patients with nonketotic hyperglycinemia.
Ann. Clin. Res. 2: (1970) 151.

Snell, K. Mitochondrial-cytosolic interrelationships involved in gluconeogenesis from serine in rat liver.
FEBS Letters 55: (1975) 202.

Snell, K. Liver enzymes of serine metabolism during neonatale development of the rat.
Biochem. J. 190: (1980) 451.

Snell, K. Enzymes of serine metabolism in normal, developing and neoplastic rat tissue.
Adv. Enzyme regul. 22: (1984) 325.

Snell, K. The duality of pathways for serine biosynthesis is a fallacy.
Trends Biochem. Sic. 11: (1986) 241.

Snyder, S.H. The glycine synaptic receptor in the mammalian central nervous system.
Br. J. Pharmac. 53: (1975) 473.

Steiman, G.S., Yodkoff, M., Berman, P.H., Blazer-Yost, B. & Segal, S.S. Late-onset nonketotic hyperglycinemia and spinocerebellar degeneration.
J. Pediat. 94: (1979) 907.

Sugimoto, E., Kitagawa, Y., Nakanishi, K. & Chiba, H. Purification and properties of beef liver D-glycerate dehydrogenase.
J. Biochem. 72: (1972) 1307.

Sweetman, L., Weyler, W., Nyhan, W.L., de Cespedes, C., Loria, A. R. & Estrada, Y. Abnormal metabolites of isoleucine in a patient with propionyl-CoA carboxylase deficiency.
Biomedical Mass Spectrometry 5: (1978)198.

Tada, T., Corbeel, L.M., Eeckers, R. & Eggermont, E. A block in glycine cleavage reaction as a common mechanism in ketotic and nonketotic hyperglycinemia.
Pediat. Res. 8: (1974) 721.

Tada, K., Narisawa, K., Yoshida, T., Konno, T., Yokoyama, Y., Nakagawa, H., Tanno, K., Mochizuki, K., Arakawa, T. & Kikuchi, G. Hyperglycinemia: A defect in glycine cleavage reaction.
Tohoku J. Exp. Med. 98: (1969) 289.

Tada, K., Yoshida, T., Morikawa, T., Minakawa, A., Wada, Y., Ando, T. & Shimura, K. Idiopathic hyperglycinemia.
Tohoku J. Exp. Med. 80: (1963) 218.

Tanaka, K., Budd, M.A., Efron, M.L. & Isselbacher, K.J. Isovaleric acidemia: A new genetic defect of leucine metabolism.
Proc. Natl. Acad. Sci. USA 56: (1966) 236.

Thieden, H.I.D., Grunnet, N., Damgaard, S.E. & Sestoft, F. Effect of fructose and glyceraldehyde on ethanol metabolism in human liver and in rat liver.
Eur. J. Biochem. 30: (1972) 250.

Trijbels, J.M.F., Monnens, L.A.H., van der Zee, S.P.M., Vrenken, J.A.T., Sengers, R.C.A. & Schretlen, E.D.A.M. A patient with nonketotic hyperglycinemia: Biochemical findings and therapeutic approaches.
Pediat. Res. 8: (1974) 598.

Truscott, R.J.W., Hick, L., Pullin, C., Halpern, B. Wilcken, B., Griffiths, H., Silink, M., Kilham, H. & Grunseit, F. Dicarboxylic aciduria: The response to fasting.
Clin.Chim. Acta 94: (1979) 31.

Uhr, M.L. Glycine decarboxylation in the central nervous system.
J. Neurochem. 20: (1973) 1005.

Van den Berghe, G. Biochemical aspects of hereditary fructose intolerance. in Hommes, F.A. and Van der Berghe, C.J., (eds.). Normal and pathological development of energy metabolism.
Academic press, London, 1975. p 211.

Von Wendt, L. Nonketotic hyperglycinemia. A clinical and experimental study. Acta Univ. Oul. D 53. Med. Interna Pædiatr. 8: (1980) 1.

Von Wendt, L. & Similä, S. Experience with nonketotic hyperglycinemia in Finland.
J. Inher. Metab. Dis. 5: (1982) 111.

Von Wendt, L., Similä, S., Saukkonen, A.L., Koivisto, M. & Kouvalainen, K. Prenatal brain damage in nonketotic hyperglycinemia.
Am. J. Dis. Child, 135: (1981) 1072.

Wadman, S.K., Duran, M., Ketting, D., Bruinvis, L., de Bree, P.K., Kamerling, J.P., Gerwig, G.J., Vliegenthart, J.F.G., Przyrembel, H., Becker, K. & Bremer, H.J. D-glyceric acidemia in a patient with chronic metabolic acidosis.
Clin. Chim. Acta 71: (1976) 477.

Walsh, D.A. & Sallach, H.J. Comparative studies on the pathways for serine biosynthesis in animal tissues.
J. Biol. Chem. 241: (1966) 4068.

Webster, L.T., Siddiqui, U.A., Lacas, S.V., Strong, J.M. & Nieyal, J.J. Identification of separate acyl-CoA: glycine and acyl-CoA: L-glutamine N-acyltransferase activities in mitochondrial fractions from liver of rhesus monkey and man.
J. Biol. Chem. 251: (1976) 3352.

Werman, R., Davidoff, R.A. & Aprison, M.H. Inhibitory action of glycine on spinal neurons in the cat.
J. Neurophysiol. 31: (1968) 81.

Williams, H. E. & Smith, L.H. L-glyceric aciduria. A new genetic variant of primary hyperoxaluria.
New. Engl. J. Med. 278: (1968 A) 233.

Williams, H.E. & Smith, L.H. The identification and determination of glyceric acid in human urine.
J. Lab. Clin. Med 71: (1968 B) 495.

Williams, H.E. & Smith, L.H. Hyperoxaluria in L-glyceric aciduria: Possible pathogenic mechanism.
Science 171: (1971) 390.

Winnick, T., Moring-Claesson, I. & Greenberg, D.M. Distribution of radioactive carbon among certain amino acids of liver homogenate protein, following uptake experiments with labelled glycine.
J. Biol. Chem. 175: (1948) 127.

Yoshida, T. & Kikuchi, G. Comparative study on major pathways of glycine and serine catabolism in vertebrate liver.
J. Biochem. 72: (1972) 1503.

Yoshida, Y. & Kikuchi, G. Major pathways of serine and glycine catabolism in various organs of the rat and cock.
J. Biochem. 73: (1973) 1013.

Young, A.B. & Snyder, S.H. Strychnine binding associated with glycine receptors of the central nervous system.
Proc. Nat. Acad. Sci. USA. 70: (1973) 2832.